HEART FAILURE

HEART FAILURE

Edited by

Gerald Sandler
*Consultant Physician
Barnsley District General Hospital
Barnsley, UK*

and

John Fry
*General Practitioner
Beckenham, Kent, UK*

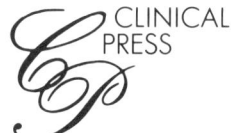

© Clinical Press Limited 1990

All rights reserved. No part of this publication may be reproduced, stored in a retrieval system, or transmitted in any form or by any means, electronic, mechanical, photocopying, recording or otherwise, without the prior permission of the Copyright Owner.

Published by Clinical Press Limited,
Redland Green Farm, Redland Green, Redland, Bristol, BS6 6HF

British Library Cataloguing in Publication Data

Heart failure. – (Clinical handbooks)
1. Man. Heart. Heart failure
I. Sandler, Gerald, 1928–
616.129

ISBN: 1-85457-008-0

Lasertypeset by Martin Lister Publishing Services, Carnforth, Lancs

Printed and bound in Great Britain by Butler & Tanner Ltd, Frome and London

Contents

Preface	vii
List of Contributors	ix
1. The pathophysiology of heart failure *D.A. Sandler*	1
2. Clinical aspects of heart failure *L.E. Ramsay*	17
3. Management of heart failure *G. Sandler*	35
4. Surgical management of heart disease *N.J. Odom and C.G.A. McGregor*	57
Index	87

Preface

Although the definition of heart failure is variable, the end result is reduced pump function of the heart and the main symptoms are breathlessness, oedema and fatigue. About 1% of the population in the United Kingdom have heart failure and 0.2% are admitted to hospital each year with this condition, so it is a common and serious problem. The prognosis is poor – 50% will die within 3 to 5 years, and if patients in New York Heart Association Class IV are considered, a half will die within 6 months to a year. Understanding of the pathophysiology, clinical manifestations and management of heart failure, has steadily improved over the last few years and it is the aim of the present volume to bring this new knowledge and understanding to the general practitioner in as clear, concise, and helpful manner as possible.

Dr David Sandler starts by discussing factors influencing cardiac function and stresses the role of the autonomic nervous system, calcium ions, the renin/angiotensin system and the atrial natriuretic hormone. He goes on to relate the causes of heart failure to alterations in the preload, afterload and myocardial contractility, and then discusses the compensatory mechanisms in heart failure, such as the neurohormonal and autonomic responses. He points out how these compensatory mechanisms lead to various clinical manifestations in heart failure.

Dr Gerald Sandler, his father, discusses the clinical aspects of heart failure. He starts with a useful clinical definition, followed by an analysis of the causes of heart failure based on intrinsic disease

PREFACE

excessive workload and increased resistance. The old concepts of forward and backward failure are discussed and then the various symptoms and signs of left and right ventricular failure detailed. The value and limitations of laboratory investigations, radiology, electrocardiography, echocardiography, radionuclide studies, cardiac catheterization and endomyocardial biopsy are considered, and he ends with some useful practical points in the diagnosis of heart failure.

The medical management of heart failure is then considered by Dr Larry Ramsay. After a brief preliminary review of the diagnosis and causes of heart failure, he considers the aims and principles of drug treatment and then goes into detailed discussion of the mainstay of treatment of heart failure, diuretics, including both benefits and problems. He then goes on to discuss the role of vasodilators in heart failure, including the angiotensin converting enzyme inhibitors, and finishes with consideration of digoxin. He supplies a very useful table summary of "stepped" treatment of heart failure.

The final chapter on surgical management of heart disease is written by two very experienced cardiac surgeons, Chris McGregor and Nicholas Odom. They first consider ischaemic heart disease and coronary bypass surgery and then go on to discuss the modern surgical approach to valvular heart disease. They finish with a detailed consideration of the very topical and important subject of cardiac transplantation. They conclude by stressing the importance of considering surgery in the earlier stages of the disease process before irreversible damage has occurred.

It is hoped that this book will help its readers to understand better the pathophysiology of heart failure which will inevitably improve the diagnosis of the condition. Rational medical therapy will then usually follow, as discussed by Dr Ramsay, but the possibility and potential of early surgical treatment should always be kept in mind, especially when limited benefit only is obtained with full medical treatment

Gerald Sandler
John Fry

List of Contributors

Christopher G.A. McGregor, MB, FRCS
Director of Cardiothoracic
 Transplantation
Mayo Clinic
Rochester
Minnesota
USA

Nicholas J. Odom, MB, FRCS
Consultant Cardiothoracic Surgeon
Royal Infirmary
Manchester
UK

Lawrence E. Ramsay, MB, ChB, FRCP
Consultant Physician
Reader in Clinical Pharmacology and
 Therapeutics
Royal Hallamshire Hospital
Sheffield
UK

David A. Sandler, MD, MRCP
Lecturer in Medicine
Queens Medical Centre
University Hospital
Nottingham
UK

Gerald Sandler, MD, FRCP
Consultant Physician
District General Hospital
Barnsley
S. Yorkshire
UK

1 The pathophysiology of heart failure

D.A. Sandler

DEFINITION OF HEART FAILURE

Heart failure is a collection of clinical features that are easily recognized. It is the state when, for whatever cause, the heart fails to perform its function of supplying an adequate amount of oxygenated blood to the tissues and organs. Consequently these tissues and organs cannot perform their function.

To understand the haemodynamic disorders in heart failure, it would be helpful to briefly review the normal physiology of the heart.

NORMAL PHYSIOLOGY OF THE HEART

Cardiac output

The cardiac output is the volume of blood in litres, which is ejected from the heart in one minute, and is the product of the heart rate and the stroke volume.

CARDIAC OUTPUT (litres/min) = HEART RATE × STROKE VOLUME

HEART FAILURE

Major factors influencing cardiac function

> PRELOAD
> AFTERLOAD
> CONTRACTILITY

These three major determinants of cardiac function also determine myocardial oxygen demand. This is particularly important in heart diseases, especially in those diseases associated with impaired coronary artery perfusion due to ischaemic heart disease.

Preload

The *preload* refers to the amount of blood in the ventricles at the end of diastole; it causes stretching of myocardial fibres, and the amount of stretch is directly related to the oxygen requirements of the heart. The healthy heart does not empty completely with each cardiac cycle so the residual blood at the end of systole forms part of the preload, added to the blood received from the atrium in diastole. An increased volume of venous blood returning to the heart will cause this preload to increase, and a healthy heart will increase the stroke volume accordingly (Frank–Starling Law).

Afterload

The *afterload* refers to the amount of resistance the ventricle has to overcome during systole. This resistance to contraction (sometimes called the impedance) is mainly determined by the peripheral arteriolar resistance, which in turn is determined by the state of vasoconstriction of the arterioles. Pathological conditions causing obstruction to flow from the heart, e.g. aortic valve stenosis, will also increase afterload.

PATHOPHYSIOLOGY OF HEART FAILURE

Contractility

Myocardial contractility is the third major determinant of cardiac function. It refers to the strength with which the myocardium contracts. Myocardial disease will often reduce the contractility of the heart. Activation of the sympathetic nervous system, for whatever reason, will increase myocardial contractility and, therefore, increase myocardial oxygen consumption.

We may now summarize the factors regulating the cardiac output:

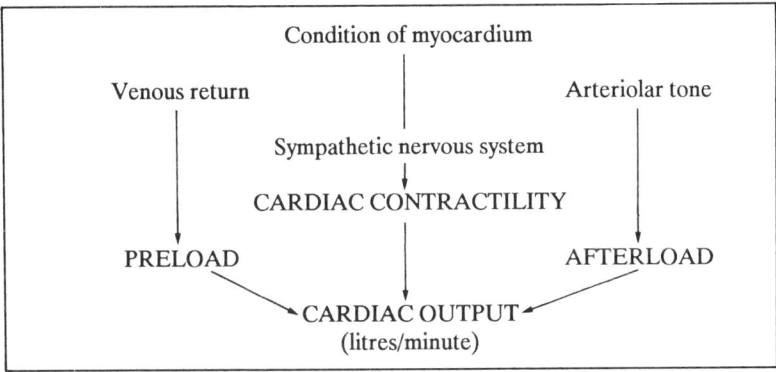

REGULATION OF NORMAL CARDIAC FUNCTION

The regulation of cardiac function is a complex combination of physiological, autonomic neurological and endocrine responses that compensate for changes in the circulation. These will be briefly mentioned here, and later they will be put into context in relation to heart failure.

FACTORS REGULATING CARDIAC FUNCTION

PHYSIOLOGICAL
AUTONOMIC
NEUROHORMONAL

HEART FAILURE

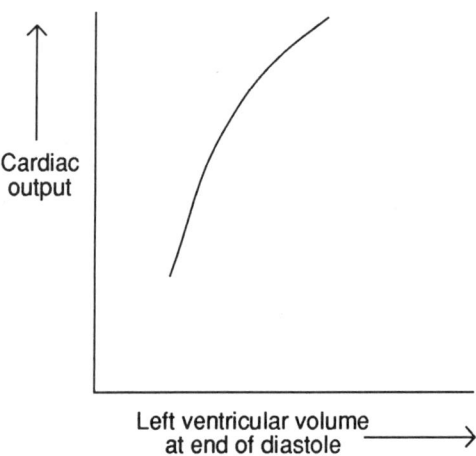

Figure 1.1 Diagrammatic representation of the curvilinear relationship between ventricular volume and cardiac output, described by Frank and Starling

Physiological

Frank–Starling law

At the turn of the century, Frank and Starling described the relationship between the end-diastolic pressure in the heart and the cardiac output and this is illustrated in Figure 1.1. This indicated that as the left ventricle filled with blood and the myocardial cells stretched, the cardiac output increased in proportion to the volume of blood within the ventricle.

Autonomic

EFFECTS OF AUTONOMIC STIMULATION ON THE HEART

PARASYMPATHETIC
- reduces heart rate (SA node)
- slows conduction through AV node
- slows ventricular conduction

SYMPATHETIC
- increases heart rate (SA node)
- increases conduction through AV node and ventricle
- increases myocardial contractility

Both the sympathetic and parasympathetic nervous systems innervate the heart. The *parasympathetic* nerves run in the vagus nerve and supply the atrial conducting system; when stimulated, acetylcholine is released which reduces sino–atrial node rate and slows conduction through the atrio–ventricular node as well as in the ventricle itself.

There are receptors in the heart which respond to the transmitters released by the *sympathetic* nervous system and they are either α or β receptors. The predominant transmitter is noradrenalin and on release it stimulates the β receptors to release further noradrenalin. This noradrenalin release stimulates the sino–atrial node to increase the heart rate, and it also accelerates the flow of calcium ions into the myocardial cells thereby increasing the contractility of this accelerated heart. Once all the β receptors available have been activated, the noradrenalin binds to α receptors and inhibits the release of further transmitter substances by a negative feedback mechanism. The effects of sympathetic stimulation of the heart are reinforced by the release of adrenalin from the adrenal gland.

Calcium and cardiac contractility

Calcium ions are important for muscular contraction. The electrical stimulus to the muscle-cell membranes result in the flow of calcium ions into the muscle cell through so-called 'slow channels'. Once the intracellular enzyme ATPase comes into contact with free calcium ions within the muscle cells, the breakdown of ATP and the release of the energy necessary for the muscular contraction can occur. One of the effects of sympathetic stimulation of myocardial cells is the increased flow of calcium through these slow channels, and thereby an increase in myocardial contractility.

Neurohormonal

Renin–angiotensin system

The *renin–angiotensin–aldosterone* axis is of major importance in the regulation of the heart and circulation. Figure 1.2 is a schematic representation of this system. The zona glomerulosa in the kidneys is very sensitive to changes in the flow of blood into the renal arterioles, and if this is reduced, renin is released, which acts on a liver substance to produce angiotensin I. This is changed by angiotensin-converting enzyme to angiotensin II, which has a dual action. It is potent *vasoconstrictor* and it causes the *release of aldosterone* from the adrenal cortex. The vasoconstriction is responsible for the diversion of blood to important organs to maintain their circulation, and aldosterone acts on the kidneys to increase the reabsorption of sodium and water, so that the circulating blood volume is increased. The combination of sodium and water conservation and vasoconstriction increases venous return to the heart and directs blood away from 'less important' tissues, such as muscle, bowel and skin, in order to maintain circulation to important organs such as heart, brain and kidneys. This compensatory mechanism is satisfactory for loss of circulating blood volume after severe haemorrhage, but has harmful effects for the failing heart.

PATHOPHYSIOLOGY OF HEART FAILURE

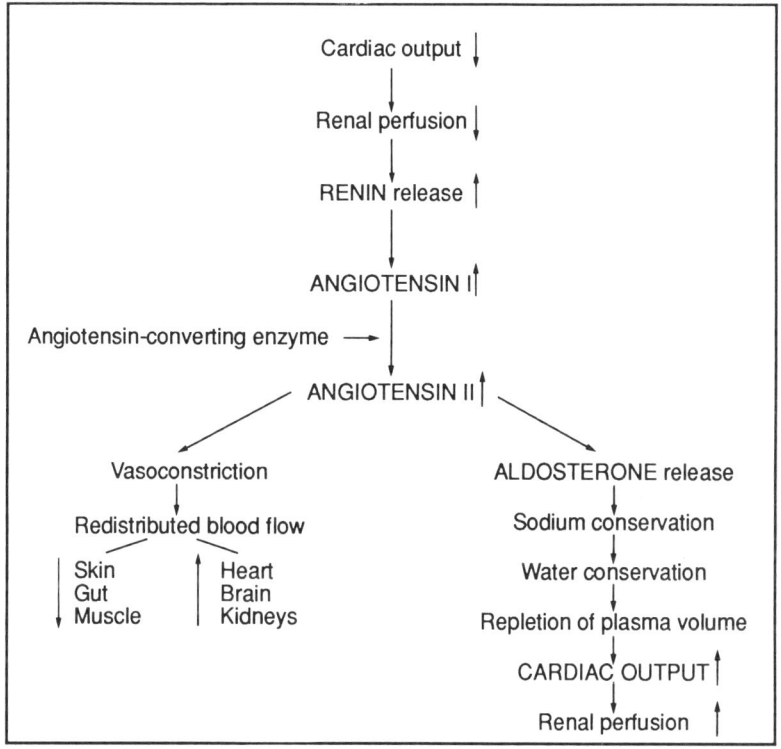

Figure 1.2 The renin–angiotensin feedback loop acting appropriately to replenish reduced blood volume

Atrial natriuretic hormone

This is a recently described hormone that is secreted by cells of the atria of the heart and circulates in the blood. It is thought that the stimulus to its secretion in hypervolaemic states is the stretching of the atrial wall due to excessive circulating blood. This peptide has been shown in experimental animals to increase glomerular filtration, and so enhance sodium excretion, to reduce the pressure in the systemic arteries and to inhibit the release of both renin and aldosterone. Heart rate and sympathetic activity have also been

HEART FAILURE

increased in these animals. These theoretical and experimental actions directly oppose the renin–angiotensin system, but their physiological role has yet to be defined.

CAUSES OF CARDIAC FAILURE

Increased preload

Factors that will increase *preload*, and so result in a volume overload for the failing heart are shown in the table below.

CAUSES OF INCREASED PRELOAD

valvular heart disease
- aortic regurgitation
- mitral regurgitation
- pulmonary regurgitation
- tricuspid regurgitation

left-to-right heart shunting
- ventricular septal defect
- atrial septal defect

excessive circulating blood volume
- over transfusion
- renin–angiotensin over-compensation

Increased afterload

Causes of increased *afterload*, or increased pressure against which the ventricle has to contract are shown in the table below.

CAUSES OF INCREASED AFTERLOAD

organic obstruction to outflow of ventricle
    left ventricle   – aortic stenosis
                              – hypertrophic obstructive cardiomyopathy
    right ventricle   – pulmonary stenosis

increased resistance due to arterial disease
    left ventricle   – hypertension
                              – coarctation of the aorta
    right ventricle   – pulmonary hypertension

PATHOPHYSIOLOGY OF HEART FAILURE

Reduced contractility of the heart

Myocardial contraction will be reduced by many diseases such as the ones illustrated in the following table.

DISEASES REDUCING CARDIAC CONTRACTILITY
- ischaemic heart disease
- cardiomyopathy
- myocarditis

Other conditions which may cause heart failure

Impaired ventricular filling

If the left ventricle is unable to fill adequately, this will result in a fall in the cardiac output, and in severe cases, heart failure; e.g. cardiac tamponade, due to excess fluid or blood in the pericardial sac. Conditions which impair ventricular filling are included in the table.

CONDITIONS IMPAIRING VENTRICULAR FILLING
- cardiac tamponade
- pericarditis (particularly constrictive)
- infiltrative myocardial diseases

Disorders of cardiac rhythm

Although the myocardium may be normal, any disorder of cardiac rhythm may impair cardiac function. A tachycardia, which may itself be due to any of the diseases mentioned above, may precipitate heart failure by the following mechanisms as shown in the table.

MECHANISMS BY WHICH TACHYDYSRHYTHMIAS MAY CAUSE HEART FAILURE
- reducing diastolic ventricular filling time, so leading to a fall in cardiac output
- increasing cardiac work and, therefore, oxygen requirements
- reducing coronary artery filling time, which occurs mainly during diastole, so impairing the function of the myocardial cells

Similarly, profound bradycardia may result in a fall in cardiac output in a diseased or damaged heart because it is unable to compensate for the reduction in heart rate by increasing the stroke volume.

WHEN THINGS GO WRONG: COMPENSATORY MECHANISMS

The compensatory mechanisms which come into play when the heart starts to fail are discussed below.

COMPENSATORY MECHANISMS IN HEART FAILURE
- cardiac dilatation
- activation of the sympathetic nervous system
- activation of the renin–angiotensin system
- cardiac hypertrophy

Cardiac dilatation

This is the first compensatory mechanism that tries to correct cardiac failure. The cardiac output can be maintained by increasing the stroke volume, and this can be achieved by increasing the amount of blood in the ventricle by cardiac dilatation. The ventricle is stretched in response to increased blood volume, so the Frank–Starling law comes into operation. Figure 1.3 shows what happens in a normal heart and also what happens in a diseased, and therefore failing, heart. Disease of the left ventricle causes a shift of the

PATHOPHYSIOLOGY OF HEART FAILURE

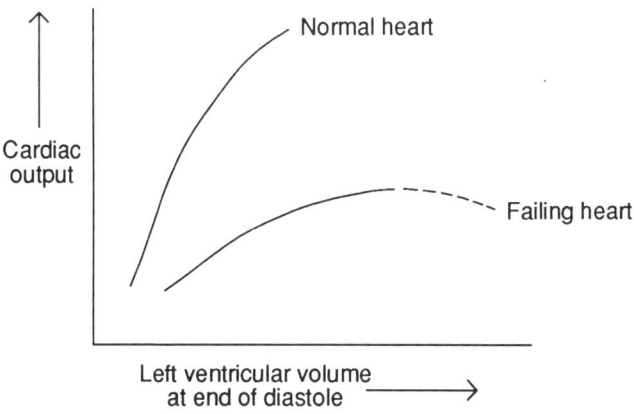

Figure 1.3 The relationship between the end-diastolic volume and the cardiac output in a normal and a failing heart

Starling curve down and to the right. This means that the increase in cardiac output in response to increased ventricular end-diastolic volume and pressure is reduced, and once a critical point of stretching is reached, the failing heart is unable to increase the cardiac output at all, so the Frank–Starling compensatory mechanism fails.

Sympathetic stimulation

Impaired cardiac output results in stimulation of the sympathetic nervous system through the β receptors of the heart. There is an increase in both the heart rate and the ventricular contractility in an effort to boost the cardiac output. At the same time, the sympathetic stimulation in the arterioles, through stimulation of their α receptors, causes a diversion of blood away from the less important tissues such as skin, muscles and bowel, towards the heart, kidneys and the brain, therefore preserving blood flow to the vital organs. Sympathetic stimulation can also affect the venous side of the circulation, and by increasing venous tone will enhance the venous return to the heart, which will increase preload in an effort to maintain cardiac output.

Neurohormonal mechanisms (renin–angiotensin system)

The renin–angiotensin mechanism takes a few days to become fully effective. An increase in angiotensin II produces vasoconstriction and diversion of blood to vital organs, and the stimulation of aldosterone release by angiotensin II increases sodium and water retention and therefore circulating blood volume; this in turn enhances venous return, so increasing the preload once again with the aim of increasing cardiac output.

Cardiac hypertrophy

This is a compensatory mechanism which takes a long time to develop. The response of the cardiac muscle cells to a persistent rise in pressure and tension within the walls of the ventricle over a number of months is to hypertrophy, so increasing the strength of overall myocardial contraction. This effect will be limited by the ability of the blood supply to the myocardium to support the hypertrophying muscle, and as the heart fails more, the myocardial oxygen supply diminishes and there is reduced ability to hypertrophy. This compensatory mechanism is 'costly' to the heart, because the increased mass of hypertrophied muscle needs a greater amount of oxygen than normal muscle to function adequately. This is neither desirable nor easily obtained in a failing heart.

CLINICAL MANIFESTATIONS OF PATHOPHYSIOLOGICAL RESPONSES IN HEART FAILURE

Heart failure may affect either the left ventricle or the right ventricle, or both (biventricular failure). The term 'congestive cardiac failure'should be avoided since there is often confusion about its meaning. Some cardiologists, especially in the United States, take this to mean left ventricular failure, but in the United Kingdom the standard interpretation is right ventricular failure. If the term 'congestive cardiac failure' is to be used, the ventricle or ventricles involved should be specified.

The clinical consequences of heart failure are shown in the table.

THE CLINICAL FEATURES OF HEART FAILURE

Low cardiac output
Sympathetic stimulation
Ventricular failure – left and/or right

Low cardiac output

In heart failure there is initially a reduction of cardiac output on exertion only, but as the failure advances the cardiac output becomes progressively poorer until it is even inadequate with the patient at rest. The manifestations of low cardiac output are summarized in the table below.

MANIFESTATIONS OF LOW CARDIAC OUTPUT
- malaise
- lethargy
- peripheral cyanosis
- reduced urine production
- poor exercise tolerance

Sympathetic overactivity

The overstimulation of the sympathetic nervous system in response to the reduced cardiac output causes vasoconstriction. The clinical features of sympathetic stimulation are shown in the following table.

HEART FAILURE

MANIFESTATIONS OF SYMPATHETIC OVERACTIVITY
- tachycardia
- cool peripheries
- sweating
- tachyarrhythmias

Congestive manifestations

Clinical manifestations of left ventricular failure

The main manifestations of left ventricular failure are:
1. Pulmonary congestion or oedema due to backpressure in the pulmonary venous circulation – this leads to breathlessness.
2. A gallop rhythm due to an additional heart sound – either a third heart sound due to an increased volume of blood entering the ventricle in early diastole, or a fourth (atrial) sound late in diastole due to forceful atrial contraction.

Gallop rhythm – 3rd heart sound (protodiastolic)

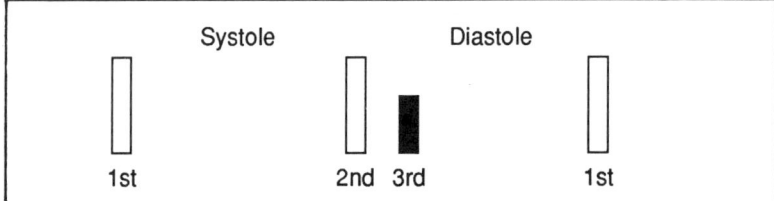

Gallop rhythm – 4th heart sound (pre-systolic)

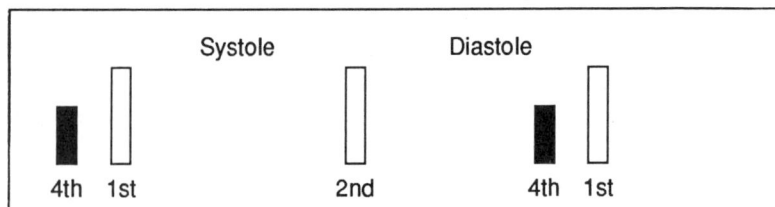

3. 'Functional' mitral regurgitation due to dilatation of the valve ring following left ventricular dilatation – this causes a systolic murmur.

4. A pleural effusion may occur sometimes, usually left-sided.

Clinical manifestations of right ventricular failure

These are due predominantly to back pressure in the systemic venous circulation and include:

- distension of neck veins
- hepatic congestion
- dependent oedema
- ascites if heart failure is severe or prolonged
- pleural effusion sometimes, usually right-sided
- systolic murmur of tricuspid incompetence occasionally
- a gallop rhythm may also be heard – this is usually due to a 3rd heart sound.

Conclusion

The function of the normal heart is controlled by a number of physiological mechanisms. When a diseased heart begins to fail, the physiological mechanisms can compensate for the impaired cardiac function up to a point, but then the cardiac disease progresses and these compensatory mechanisms can no longer improve the situation. At this stage, the clinical manifestations of cardiac failure become apparent.

2 Clinical aspects of heart failure

G. Sandler

DEFINITION

There are a variety of ways of defining heart failure. A useful clinical definition is:

A failure of the heart to meet the varying metabolic and oxygen needs of the body.

In haemodynamic terms, this means that when heart failure is present there is increased end-diastolic ventricular volume and pressure with a decreased cardiac output on exercise, or in more severe cases, at rest also.

CAUSES OF HEART FAILURE

The heart may fail either as a result of intrinsic disease or because of excessive workload.

Intrinsic disease

- ischaemic heart disease – commonest cause

HEART FAILURE

- cardiomyopathy (dilated)
- myocarditis from whatever cause
- myocardial infiltration
  - amyloid
  - sarcoid
  - haemachromatosis

Excessive workload

This may be in the form of either increased resistance for the heart to overcome (pressure load), increased volume of blood for the heart to expel (volume overload) or a generalized increase in metabolic demands on the heart.

Increased resistance

Left ventricle	– hypertension
	– aortic stenosis
	– hypertrophic obstructive cardio-myopathy (HOCM)
Right ventricle	– chronic obstructive lung disease
	– pulmonary fibrosis
	– pulmonary stenosis
	– pulmonary thrombo-embolic disease
	– idiopathic pulmonary hypertension
Increased volume	– aortic/mitral/tricuspid incompetence
	– atrial/ventricular septal defects with shunting
Increased demands	– thyrotoxicosis
	– anaemia
	– pregnancy
	– Paget's disease of bone
	– arteriovenous fistulae

CLINICAL ASPECTS OF HEART FAILURE

In addition to the basic underlying cause of the heart failure, the condition, which may be latent, can be precipitated by a variety of factors:

- sudden arrhythmia, either tachyarrhythmia, e.g. atrial fibrillation or bradyarrhythmia, e.g. heart block or severe sinus bradycardia
- systemic infection which produces tachycardia and increased metabolic demands
- pulmonary embolism which leads to fever, tachycardia and increased right ventricular pressure
- strenuous exertion in a weakened heart
- superimposed myocarditis
- increased metabolic demands from anaemia, thyrotoxicosis and pregnancy
- renal failure which increases sodium retention with consequent fluid overload
- inappropriate withdrawal of heart failure treatment, e.g. diuretics, salt restriction

Forward and backward failure

Traditionally, a distinction has been made between forward failure and backward failure.

The clinical manifestations of 'forward' failure are attributed to reduced perfusion of vital organs:

Brain	→	confusion
Muscles	→	weakness
Kidneys	→	sodium retention and fluid overload

'Backward' failure is regarded as being due to damming of blood behind either ventricle leading to increased transudation of fluid:

Lungs	→	dyspnoea
Subcutaneous tissues	→	oedema
Liver	→	congestion and enlargement
Peritoneal cavity	→	ascites

Since both mechanisms tend to be active in most patients with chronic heart failure, the distinction between forward and backward failure becomes less helpful diagnostically and therapeutically.

SYMPTOMS AND SIGNS OF HEART FAILURE

Left ventricular failure (Figure 2.1)

Symptoms

Breathlessness – is the cardinal symptom of left ventricular failure. The features are:

- initially only on exertion
- later at rest
- worse lying down (orthopnoea)
- in severe cases, paroxysmal nocturnal dyspnoea occurs due to attacks of pulmonary oedema
- wheezing is frequent in pulmonary oedema
- cough and haemoptysis (pink frothy sputum) may occur in pulmonary oedema

Although the mechanism of the breathlessness has traditionally been attributed to an increase in left atrial pressure leading to pulmonary venous congestion and transudation of fluid into alveoli, Lipkin and Poole–Wilson[1] are doubtful of this view, since on investigation there is no consistent relationship between breathlessness and the left atrial pressure or left ventricular function; nor is the breathlessness related to lung compliance (stiffness): the mechanism of the dyspnoea remains unknown.

CLINICAL ASPECTS OF HEART FAILURE

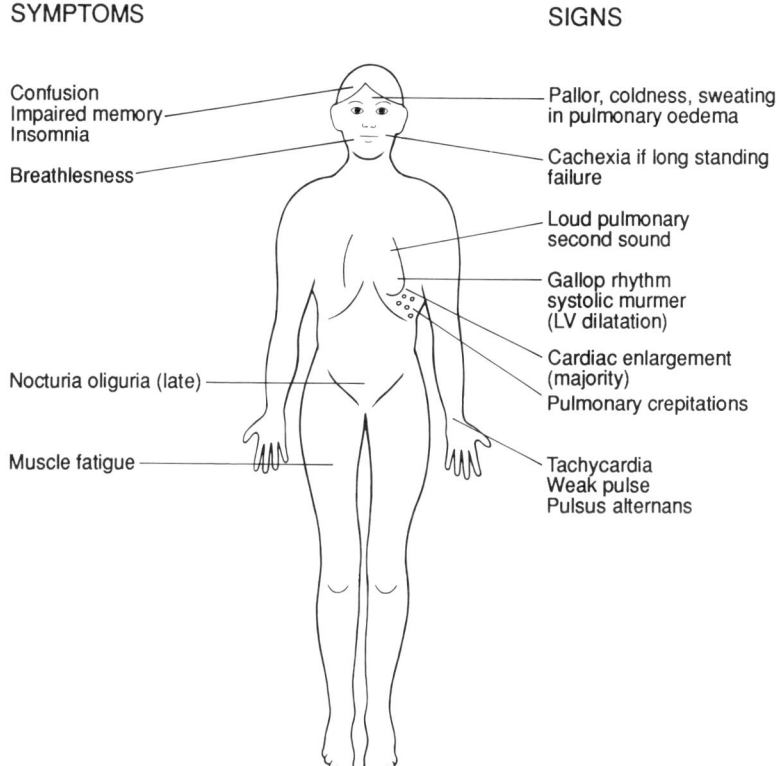

Figure 2.1 Symptoms and signs of left venticular failure

The wheezing which occurs in acute pulmonary oedema is due to congestion of the bronchial veins and bronchial mucosal oedema, and may lead to difficulty in distinguishing acute pulmonary oedema with wheezing (cardiac asthma) from true bronchial asthma. Helpful differentiating features will be discussed in the following section on examination findings in left ventricular failure (Table 2.1).

A useful simple classification of heart failure has been suggested by the *New York Heart Association*:

HEART FAILURE

Classification of heart failure

Class I	–	No limitation with ordinary physical activity
Class II	–	Comfortable at rest, symptoms with ordinary activity (dyspnoea, fatigue, palpitations, angina)
Class III	–	Comfortable at rest, symptoms on less than ordinary activity
Class IV	–	Breathless at rest, no physical activity possible without distress

Excessive fatigue on effort – may be due to:

- a low cardiac output in heart failure with impaired muscle perfusion
- inadequate oxygen content of the perfusing blood
- excessive diuretic treatment may contribute by causing fluid depletion and hypokalaemia.

Mental symptoms – impairment of memory, confusion, insomnia, nightmares are similarly attributed to impaired cerebral perfusion as a result of the reduced cardiac output in heart failure.

Urinary symptoms – nocturia is common, and is due to increased renal perfusion in recumbency following relaxation of the compensatory renal vasoconstriction occurring in the daytime. Oliguria may be a late symptom due to renal failure.

Signs of left ventricular failure

1. *General*
- orthopnoea/dyspnoea may be evident
- peripheral cyanosis if the cardiac output is markedly reduced
- cyanotic malar flush may occur in chronic left ventricular failure from whatever cause, but is particularly likely in severe mitral valve disease
- there may be signs of marked sympathetic overactivity if pulmonary oedema is present – pallor, coldness, sweating, dilated pupils, anxiety.

CLINICAL ASPECTS OF HEART FAILURE

2. *Cardiovascular*
- pulse
  - tachycardia
  - weak due to low cardiac output
  - alternating weak and strong beats may be felt in severe cases
- blood pressure
  - may be low
  - may be high in acute pulmonary oedema due to compensatory vasoconstriction
  - pulsus alternans best detected with blood pressure – heart rate doubles as sphygmomanometer cuff is deflated
- apex beat
  - displaced to left due to cardiac dilatation
  - impulse may be thrusting due to LV hypertrophy (e.g. hypertensive)
- heart sounds
  - often muffled
  - a gallop rhythm is frequent – due to a 3rd or 4th sound
  - a 3rd heart sound is more indicative of heart failure, either left or right; a 4th heart sound may occur in left ventricular failure but also in left ventricular strain without failure, e.g. in hypertension
  - if the heart rate is fast a summation gallop can occur when both the 3rd and 4th heart sounds are superimposed on each other
- murmurs
  - due to underlying valve disease
  - soft apical systolic murmur due to functional mitral incompetence resulting from LV dilatation
- lungs
  - fine crepitations best heard posteriorly at the lung bases – may extend upwards with more extensive pulmonary congestion
  - rhonchi due to bronchial mucosal congestion especially in acute pulmonary oedema
  - pleural effusion may occur – due to impairment of pulmonary venous and lymphatic drainage

Table 2.1 Differentiation between 'cardiac' and 'bronchial' asthma

	Cardiac	Bronchial
Past History	hypertension ischaemic heart disease valvular disease	asthma recurrent bronchitis allergy
Smoking	possible	frequent
Onset	rapid	more gradual
Timing	any time in night	often early morning
Dyspnoea	mainly inspiratory	mainly expiratory
Cough	follows dyspnoea	precedes dyspnoea
Sputum	pink, frothy	thick, gelatinous
Relief	standing up diuretic	coughing up sputum bronchodilator
Lung signs	mainly crepitations	mainly rhonchi
Cardiac signs	gallop rhythm	nil significant

Right Ventricular Failure (Figure 2.2)

Symptoms

Breathlessness – is not a prominent symptom unless:

- the RV failure is secondary to chronic LV failure
- it is due to chronic lung disease
- pleural effusion is present

Excessive fatigue may occur for similar reasons to left ventricular failure:

- inadequate perfusion of the muscles
- impaired oxygen content of the blood
- an additional factor may be blood volume depletion and hypokalaemia due to intensive diuretic treatment
- poor appetite and poor food intake due to the hepatic and intestinal congestion, or to drug toxicity, may also contribute to the weakness.

CLINICAL ASPECTS OF HEART FAILURE

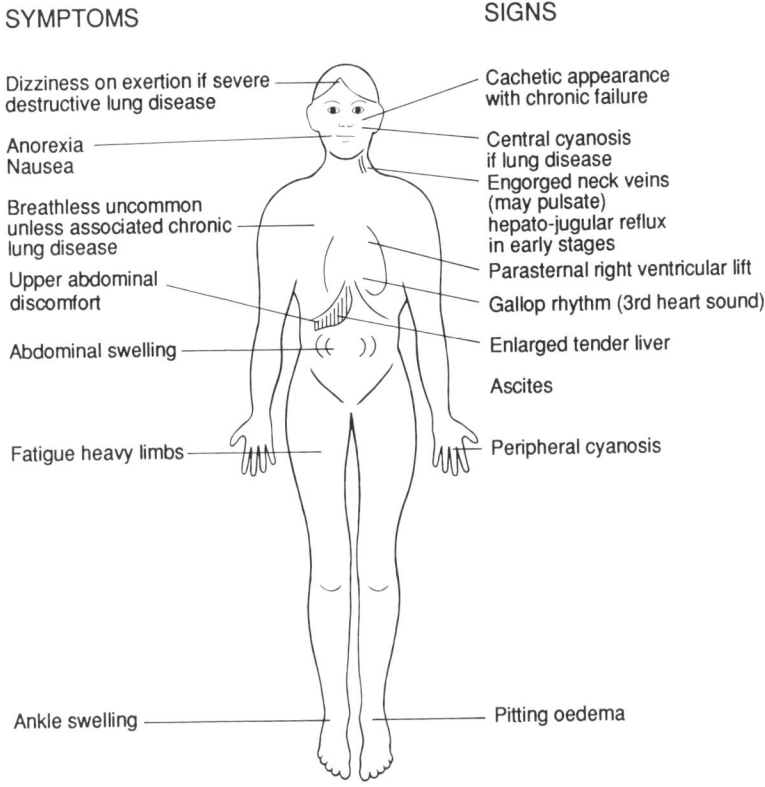

Figure 2.2 Symptoms and signs of right ventricular failure

Gastrointestinal
- upper abdominal pain and tenderness due to congestion of the liver
- anorexia, nausea, fullness after meals, constipation due to congestion of the GI tract
- diarrhoea may occur in severe cases associated with malabsorption.

Swelling of feet due to oedema.

HEART FAILURE

Swelling of abdomen due to ascites.

Dizziness/syncope may occur on effort when right heart failure is due to severe chronic obstructive lung disease.

Weight gain due to oedema.

Signs

Cyanosis is often present due to venous stagnation.

Oedema. This occurs in the dependent parts – ankles and feet if ambulant, and sacral area if bedridden. In severe cases, generalized oedema may occur (anasarca).

Neck veins will be distended due to an increase in systemic venous pressure. If functional tricuspid incompetence occurs the neck veins may be pulsatile with giant 'V' waves.

Hepatomegaly – The liver will be enlarged, firm and tender, in the acute situation. Long-standing right ventricular failure may lead to a chronically enlarged, firm, non-tender, liver due to cardiac 'cirrhosis'.

Jaundice may occur as a result of hepatic congestion and especially if cardiac 'cirrhosis' is present.

Ascites may occur in severe cases.

Cardiac findings

- tachycardia often with full volume pulse ('high output' state)
- left parasternal lift due to right ventricular hypertrophy
- gallop due to a 3rd heart sound may be present
- loud pulmonary 2nd sound if chronic LV failure or chronic lung disease present.

Lung findings
- signs of underlying chronic lung disease if present

- pleural effusions may occur – often bilateral in right ventricular failure.

Cachexia – often occurs in long-standing right ventricular failure and is due to:

- hepatic/intestinal congestion
    - anorexia
    - impaired fat absorption
    - protein-losing enteropathy
- increased metabolism
    - increase in myocardial oxygen consumption
    - excessive work of breathing
    - low grade fever often present
- mental depression and drug toxicity may also contribute

INVESTIGATION IN HEART FAILURE
Laboratory tests

Urine – may show protein and granular casts indicative of renal damage as a result of the heart failure.

Blood urea/serum creatinine – may be increased as a result of reduced renal perfusion or renal damage; the distinction between the two can be based on urinary specific gravity – if it is high renal disease is unlikely.

Serum electrolytes
- normal prior to treatment
- Na^+ ↓ with diuretic/salt restriction
- K^+ ↓ with potent diuretics
- K^+ ↑ in severe heart failure – due to severely restricted glomerular filtration

Liver function tests
- enzymes increased with liver congestion – especially SGOT and alkaline phosphatase
- bilirubin increased

- prothrombin concentration may be reduced with severe liver involvement – especially 'cardiac cirrhosis'
- albumin ↑ with cardiac cirrhosis

Blood count – is usually unaltered unless there is secondary polycythaemia due to cor pulmonale.

Special laboratory tests may be necessary if specific conditions are suspected as a cause of the heart failure:
- thyrotoxicosis – thyroid function
- infective endocarditis – blood culture
- collagen disorder – collagen screen, immunophoresis
- phaeochromocytoma – blood and urinary levels of catecholamines

Radiology

Chest x-ray – this can be helpful in several ways:

Heart
- size and shape of the heart gives useful information on the nature of the underlying heart disease, e.g., 'boot-shaped' heart due to left ventricular enlargement in hypertension (Figure 2.3) or a 'ham-shaped' heart with a prominent pulmonary conus in mitral valve disease.

Lungs
- normally basal venous size is larger than apical; in left ventricular failure this is reversed (upper lobe venous congestion)
- interstitial pulmonary oedema produces lines radiating out from the hila (Kerley A lines) or peripheral horizontal lines (Kerley B lines)
- gross pulmonary oedema produces a 'butterfly' flare radiating out from the hila (Figure 2.4)
- pleural effusions may occur in severe left or right ventricular failure

Other possible findings on chest X-ray which may be relevant in causing heart failure and may be remediable include:

CLINICAL ASPECTS OF HEART FAILURE

- coarctation of aorta → rib notching
- dissecting aneurysm of aorta
- aortic valve disease → calcification
- left ventricular aneurysm
- constrictive pericarditis

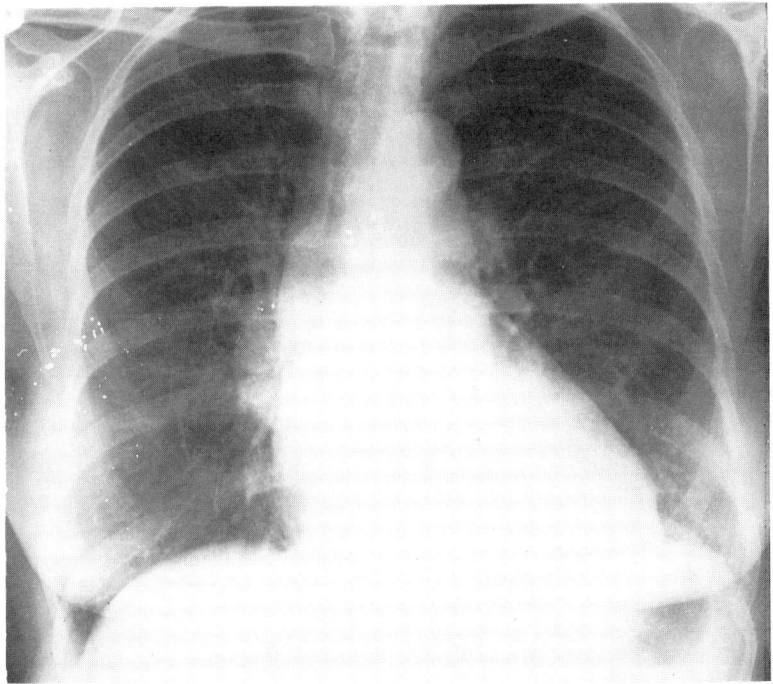

Figure 2.3 Chest X-ray showing 'boot-shaped heart' due to left ventricular enlargement in a hypertensive patient

HEART FAILURE

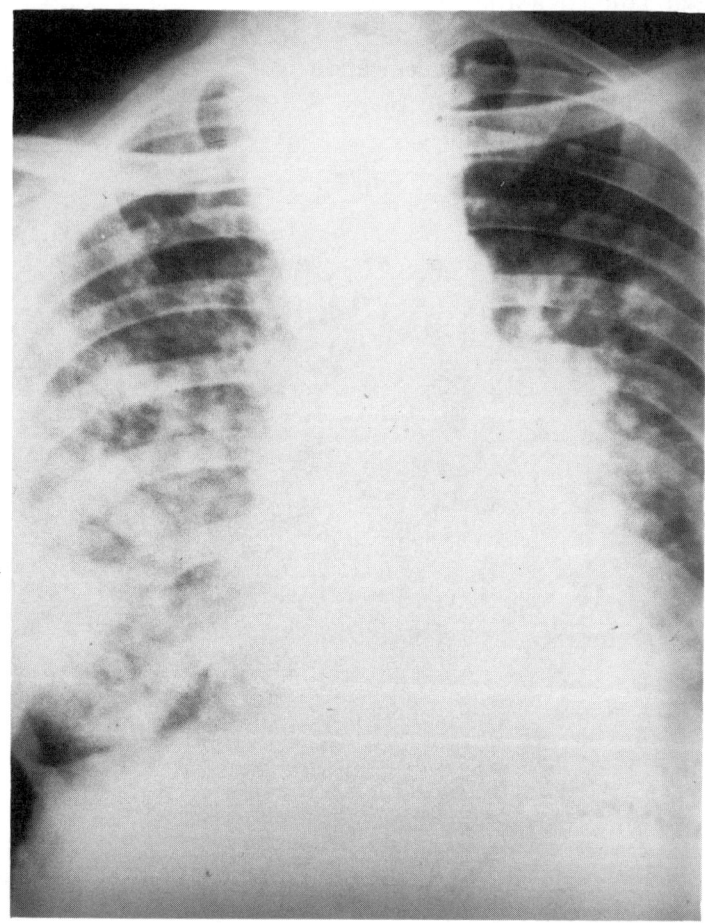

Figure 2.4 Chest X-ray showing pulmonary oedema

Electrocardiography

There are no specific changes in heart failure though the voltage of the complexes may be generally poor in chronic heart failure. The changes which may be helpful to diagnosis include:

- ischaemia – may be a cause
- arrhythmias
- bifid P wave in mitral valve disease
- left ventricular hypertrophy and strain resulting from hypertension or valvular heart disease
- right ventricular hypertrophy and strain indicating chronic parenchymatous lung disease, thrombo-embolic disease or pulmonary hypertension
- persistent S-T elevation in left ventricular aneurysm
- rarely electrical alternans may occur in severe heart failure
- digoxin toxicity and hypokalaemic changes resulting from diuretics can also be detected

Echocardiography

One-dimensional M mode or two-dimensional echocardiography can be helpful in showing structural and functional abnormalities of the heart. In particular, it can show:

- chamber size
- wall and septal thickness
- mitral and aortic valve disease
- systolic function
- ventricular compliance (ability to expand in diastole)
- regional ventricular wall motion
- left ventricular aneurysm
- left atrial myxoma
- pericardial effusion

HEART FAILURE

Radionuclide studies

Radio-isotope studies with technetium pyrophosphate and thallium can be helpful in revealing abnormalities of structure and function of the heart. Thallium is useful in showing myocardial perfusion defects in angina during an exercise test and also in established myocardial infarction. Technetium is also of value in showing ischaemic myocardium during the acute phase of myocardial infarction, but can also be used in 'gated' studies (i.e. synchronized to the electrocardiogram) to measure the left ventricular ejection fraction which is a very useful indicator of the degree of left ventricular dysfunction in heart failure. Other useful information includes diagnosis of cardiomyopathy and atrial myxoma.

Cardiac catheterization

Left side of the heart

Catheterization of the left ventricle with angiocardiography is helpful in showing the following causes of left ventricular failure

- mitral or aortic valve disease
- left ventricular aneurysm
- atrial and ventricular septal defects causing left-to-right shunts

Right side of the heart

Catheterization of the superior vena cava and right atrium with a central venous line can give helpful date in:

- diagnosis of right ventricular failure
- detection of fluid depletion (hypovolaemia)
- monitoring of infusion therapy to avoid fluid overload
- monitoring of diuretic therapy in heart failure to determine optimal treatment

CLINICAL ASPECTS OF HEART FAILURE

Catheterization of the right ventricle, pulmonary artery and pulmonary capillaries (wedge pressure) with a Swan–Ganz balloon catheter is very helpful in the diagnosis and treatment of left ventricular failure. The pulmonary wedge pressure gives an indirect measure of left atrial pressure which reflects left ventricular function.

The cardiac output and cardiac index (output/square metre of body surface) can also be measured with a Swan–Ganz catheter.

Endomyocardial biopsy

These are techniques for biopsying the endocardium and myocardium of both the right and left ventricle. It is an investigation which is available in only a few specialized cardiac centres.

It is valuable in the diagnosis of:

- cardiomyopathy
- Loeffler's endocarditis
- immunological rejection of cardiac transplant
- cardiac toxicity with cytotoxic drugs for breast cancer, e.g. adriamycin

CONCLUSIONS

The following are useful practical points in the diagnosis of heart failure:

- the diagnostic triad for left ventricular failure is:
  - dyspnoea
  - basal crepitations
  - gallop rhythm
- the diagnostic triad for right ventricular failure is:
  - distended neck veins
  - oedema
  - congestion of the liver
- the commonest cause of left ventricular failure in the UK is hypertension: the commonest cause of right ventricular failure is chronic lung disease (cor pulmonale)
- latent heart failure can be made overt by associated anaemia, thyrotoxicosis, systemic infection and arrhythmias, all of which are reversible
- severe wheezing can occur in acute pulmonary oedema and simulate acute bronchial asthma. The two conditions can usually be differentiated by a good clinical history and by the clinical signs on examination
- a chest X-ray is probably the most helpful simple test in left heart failure both in the diagnosis of the failure (changes in the lungs) and in suggesting possible causes (changes in heart size and shape).

REFERENCE

1. Lipkin, D.P. and Poole-Wilson, P.A. (1986). Symptoms limiting exercise in chronic heart failure. *Br. Med. J.*, **292**, 1030–1

3 Management of heart failure

L.E. Ramsay

INTRODUCTION

It is a never ending struggle to keep up with advances in therapeutics, and it must be doubly difficult for those in general practice who have to keep an eye on all areas of medicine. Ideas on the treatment of heart failure have altered greatly in the last 10 years. The emphasis has switched away from direct stimulation of the failing heart, hoping thus to improve its function. The new point of attack is the complex neurohumoral and haemodynamic response to impaired cardiac function – a response which is now thought to further worsen the cardiac function. Do these new ideas matter? Are the new methods of treatment a real advance, or are they merely a passing fashion in therapeutics? Fortunately the new ideas have been put to the test in soundly designed and carefully conducted controlled clinical trails. Those trials leave no doubt that modern treatment does improve symptom control in heart failure, and moreover have shown that the length of life is substantially prolonged. Those who still cling to the traditional 'digoxin and diuretic' routine are now offering their patients sub-optimal symptom relief and a shorter lifespan than could be achieved.

HEART FAILURE

DIAGNOSING HEART FAILURE

Before considering treatment, three questions have to be answered when approaching any patient with symptoms or signs suggesting heart failure.

Is it really heart failure?

Most patients with ankle swelling do *not* have heart failure. The elderly and immobile often have a local cause for oedema, and drug-induced oedema is reaching near-epidemic proportions because of the wide use of the dihydropyridine calcium antagonists such as nifedipine (Adalat) and nicardipine (Cardene). Oedema can be attributed, with confidence, to right heart failure only when all three components of the classical diagnostic triad are present – oedema, elevated jugular venous pressure and hepatomegaly – and when other causes of generalized fluid retention such as chronic liver disease and nephrotic syndrome have been excluded. It follows that the diagnosis requires an adequate history and examination, and usually a few investigations (chest X-ray, ECG, test for proteinuria and liver function tests).

Left ventricular failure may also cause diagnostic difficulty. Typical features such as exertional dyspnoea, nocturnal dyspnoea and crepitations at the lung bases are also found in chronic bronchitis, late-onset asthma and various forms of pulmonary fibrosis. In acute situations it can be difficult or impossible to tell whether a patient has bronchopneumonia, left ventricular failure or both. A chest X-ray is usually helpful, and one should be wary of the diagnosis of left ventricular failure if there is no cardiomegaly and no evidence of pulmonary venous congestion (prominent upper lobe veins, Kerley B lines, pleural transudates, alveolar shadowing of pulmonary oedema).

What is causing the failure?

The importance of this question cannot be exaggerated. When there is no correctable cause for heart failure the prognosis is daunting. Half of those with mild to moderate failure die within 3 years[1], and half of those who have symptoms at rest will die within 6 months[2]. Modern treatment has some impact upon this, as will be discussed later, but the outlook is nevertheless very poor with conservative management. It follows that no effort should be spared to diagnose the cause of heart failure, and in particular to exclude the correctable causes listed in Table 3.1. It should be noted that aortic valve disease and mitral stenosis may be entirely 'silent' when heart failure is severe, and that aortic stenosis can now be palliated by transluminal balloon valvoplasty even in elderly pa-

Table 3.1 Correctable causes of heart failure, and factors which may exacerbate heart failure

Correctable causes
- Valvular heart disease
- Hypertension
- Thyrotoxicosis
- Arrhythmias (particularly uncontrolled atrial fibrillation)
- Complete heart block
- Alcoholic cardiomyopathy
- Left ventricular aneurysm
- Thiamine deficiency
- Pericardial constriction or tamponade
- Congenital heart disease
- Arteriovenous shunts

Factors which may exacerbate heart failure
- Drug treatment:
  - beta-blockers
  - verapamil
  - non-steroidal anti-inflammatory drugs
  - steroids
  - anti-arrhythmic drugs
- Anaemia
- Obesity
- Intravenous infusion
- Acute respiratory infection

HEART FAILURE

tients. Note also that heart failure may be the only clinical manifestation of thyrotoxicosis in the elderly. One should not accept too readily a presumptive diagnosis, for example of ischaemic heart disease. If a positive diagnosis cannot be reached, the patient should be referred for detailed investigation.

Is there a precipitating factor?

Possible precipitants for a recent onset or worsening of heart failure should be sought, even when the cause of heart failure is evident. Where there has been a clear precipitant it may prove possible to withdraw or reduce anti-failure treatment at a later date. For example, most patients with heart failure soon after a myocardial infarction will not need lifelong treatment.

CHRONIC HEART FAILURE

General measures

Dyspnoea and fatigue are likely to limit physical activity appropriately, and the doctor need not impose additional restrictions. Bedrest should be avoided unless it becomes inevitable in severe resistant failure, and when it is necessary anticoagulation should be considered to reduce the high risk of venous thromboembolism. Patients should avoid added salt at table, but formal salt restriction is helpful only in resistant heart failure. Weight reduction should be advised for those who are overweight. Fluid restriction is necessary only when the serum sodium falls below 130 mmol/l.

Drug therapy

Aims

Treatment of heart failure aims to relieve the symptoms (Table 3.2) and to prolong life – hopefully life of a reasonable quality. Of the symptoms listed in Table 3.2, fatigue is often the most distressing to

MANAGEMENT OF HEART FAILURE

Table 3.2 Symptoms and signs of heart failure

	Right heart failure	Left heart failure
Symptoms:	fatigue	exertional dyspnoea
	oedema	orthopnoea
	abdominal swelling	paroxysmal dyspnoea
	anorexia	fatigue
	nausea	cough
	weight loss	haemoptysis
	epigastric pain	wheezing
	confusion	confusion
Physical signs:	ankle or sacral oedema	tachypnoea
	elevated JVP	tachycardia
	tender hepatomegaly	displaced apex beat
	displaced apex beat	pulsus alternans
	gallop rhythm	basal crepitations
	jaundice	gallop rhythm

the patient and the least appreciated by the doctor. It is commonly asserted that traditional treatment based largely on diuretics did not prolong life, but this is probably incorrect. Fulminant left ventricular failure was corrected, and water-logged patients were returned to reasonable health, by diuretic therapy, and it is inconceivable that life was not prolonged in some of these patients. Diuretics were so obviously effective that a placebo-controlled trial could never have been justified. We will see later that formal controlled trials have shown that vasodilator therapy does prolong life when it is superimposed upon diuretic treatment, but it would be quite wrong to conclude from this that vasodilator treatment is superior to diuretic treatment.

Principles of drug treatment

The neurohumoral and haemodynamic changes observed in heart failure are shown, in much-simplified form, in Figure 3.1. The details are not important – what does matter is the concept that 'compensatory increases in preload (venous return) and afterload (peripheral resistance) cause further impairment in cardiac func-

HEART FAILURE

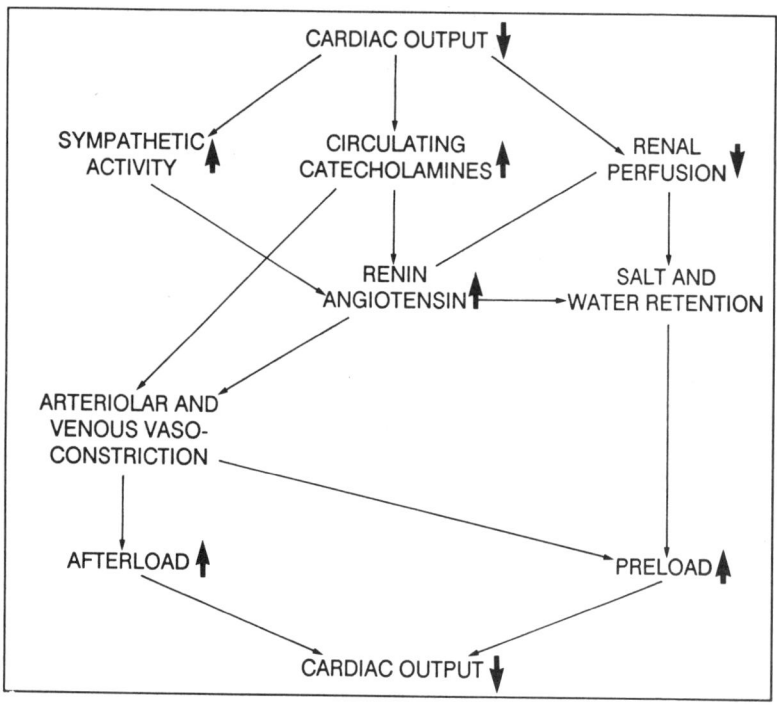

Figure 3.1 Simplified scheme of the haemodynamic and neurohumoral responses in cardiac failure

tion. In other words homeostatic responses, which initially maintain the circulatory *status quo*, become harmful, and worsen the heart failure, at some stage in the progression of the illness. The traditional therapeutic approach was to attempt to improve cardiac contractility by using inotropic agents such as digoxin. It is now clear that this has little effect upon cardiac function when the patient is in sinus rhythm, and there are indeed hints that inotropic agents may worsen the prognosis. Modern treatment aims to improve cardiac function by reducing the preload with diuretics and venodilators, and the afterload with arteriolar vasodilators. There is already ample evidence that this approach is effective both in relieving symptoms and in prolonging life.

Diuretics

General – by escalating diuretic treatment stepwise it is possible to abolish fluid retention, even in patients with the most severe heart failure, and this treatment 'ladder' will be described below. The most important unanswered question in the management of heart failure at present is exactly when to stop 'climbing' the diuretic ladder, and to add a vasodilator to the regimen. The evidence available on this point will be discussed later.

Classes of diuretic – the properties of the diuretics available are shown in Table 3.3. In practice one needs to be familiar with only three diuretics – one thiazide (bendrofluazide), one loop diuretic (frusemide) and one potassium-sparing drug (spironolactone). None of the alternatives has any real advantage, and many of them are more expensive than the drugs mentioned.

Thiazide diuretics. Thiazides have a prolonged action and a flat dose-response, and are, therefore, given once daily and without dose-titration, e.g. bendrofluazide 5 mg daily. They have only modest potency and are only suitable for mild heart failure. A loop

Table 3.3 Classes of diuretic used in heart failure

	Thiazides	*Loop diuretics*	*Potassium-sparers*
Examples	bendrofluazide	frusemide bumetanide	spironolactone amiloride triamterene
Administration	oral	oral or i.v.	oral
Dose-response	flat	steep	flat
Duration	12–72 hours	4–6 hours	24 hours
Potency	moderate	high	weak
Contraindications	gout diabetes renal failure	gout diabetes prostatism	renal failure
Interactions	lithium	lithium aminoglycosides cephalosporins	potassium ACE inhibitors

ACE – Angiotensin converting enzyme

diuretic should be chosen when failure is severe or needs urgent treatment. The thiazides have three advantages over the loop diuretics when the failure is mild; the diuresis is less brisk and less socially disruptive; they have a superior anti-hypertensive effect when there is coexistent hypertension; and they are less expensive. On the other hand they occasionally cause troublesome nocturia, and they are ineffective in advanced renal failure. The side-effects of thiazides (and loop diuretics) are shown in Table 3.4. Most of

Table 3.4 Side-effects of thiazide and loop diuretics

Subjective	Biochemical
Skin rashes	Hypokalaemia
Acute gout	Hyperuricaemia
Diabetes	Hyponatraemia
Impotence	Glucose intolerance
Urinary retention	Hyperlipidaemia
Loin pain	Hypomagnesaemia
Purpura	Hypercalcaemia (thiazides only)
Acute pancreatitis	

them are biochemical phenomena which do not trouble patients, and despite the fuss made about them in recent years they are probably harmless. The evidence that the benefits of thiazide treatment outweigh any theoretical risk is now incontrovertible. In practice the main problems are occasional instances of gout and diabetes. The question of hypokalaemia is discussed below.

Loop diuretics. Frusemide has a short (4–6 hour) and brisk diuretic action which occasionally precipitates urinary retention in elderly men. Despite its short action it is effective when given once daily. It is the drug of choice for heart failure which is severe or requires urgent treatment. The dose-response is steep, and the dose should be increased stepwise from 40 mg daily until the desired response is attained. Doses as high as 1–2 g daily are required in special circumstances, but in practice one would consider adding vasodilator therapy when a daily dose higher than 120–250 mg is needed (see below). Loop diuretics remain effective in advanced renal failure.

Potassium problems. there can be few areas of medical practice in which doctors' beliefs and prescribing habits are so much at odds with the established facts. These facts are as follows:

1. Thiazide and loop diuretics do not cause potassium *depletion*. They do cause *hypokalaemia*, with no important fall in intracellular potassium, and the cause is a sustained increase in the renal clearance of potassium. Potassium supplements cannot correct this, and even daily doses as high as 64 mmol potassium chloride (e.g. eight slow k tablets) will not abolish diuretic-induced hypokalaemia. The small doses of potassium chloride in combined tablets such as Neo-Naclex K, kavidrex K, kurinex K, etc. have no measurable effect on serum potassium. They should *not* be prescribed. When diuretic-induced hypokalaemia does need to be prevented or treated one of the potassium-sparing diuretics described below should be used. These drugs reduce the renal clearance of potassium and, if the correct dose is used, abolish hypokalaemia.
2. Increased dietary potassium will *not* prevent or correct diuretic-induced hypokalaemia. Potassium in the diet is not more effective than potassium in tablets, and patients would have to drink litres of fruit juice or eat metres of banana to get any useful effect. If potassium *was* effective it would be cheaper and more convenient to take potassium chloride tablets.
3. Loop diuretics such as frusemide do *not* cause more severe hypokalaemia than the thiazides – the opposite is the case. Thiazides lower serum potassium[3] by an average of 0.6 mmol/l, loop diuretics by only 0.3 mmol/l.
4. Patients with heart failure are *not* more likely to become hypokalaemic with diuretics – they are less likely than hypertensive subjects to become hypokalaemic.[3] Serum potassium is actually elevated, by a mean of 0.5 mmol/l, in untreated heart failure, and diuretic treatment returns it to the 'normal' level on average.

HEART FAILURE

5. Elderly patients are *not* more likely to become hypokalaemic on diuretic treatment – the opposite is the case.[3]
6. Mild hypokalaemia does *not* cause any symptoms. Symptoms occur only when the serum potassium falls to levels of 2.5 mmol/l or lower – levels very rarely observed during diuretic treatment.
7. Diuretic-induced hypokalaemia is *not progressive*. The serum potassium falls over 1 or 2 weeks, and then remains constant over long periods of time unless the dose of diuretic is altered.
8. Mild hypokalaemia (3.0–3.5 mmol/l) does *not* cause clinically significant arrhythmias in the vast majority of patients. However it may be dangerous, and must be avoided, in a minority of patients who have additional problems. Patients at risk are shown in Table 2.5.

Table 3.5 Situations in which diuretic-induced hypokalaemia should be prevented or corrected

- Digoxin treatment
- Drugs which prolong the Q–T interval: prenylamine, sotalol, quinidine, amiodarone, other antiarrhythmics
- History of paroxysmal arrhythmias
- Severe or unstable angina
- Co-existent chronic liver disease
- Severe hypokalaemia: < 3.0 mmol/l

What are the practical implications of these points? Those patients who are at risk from any degree of hypokalaemia (Table 3.5) must be identified, and should have effective prophylaxis against hypokalaemia from the start of treatment. This involves co-prescription of a potassium-sparing drug (*not* potassium supplements) with the thiazide or loop diuretic from the outset. This does not guarantee normokalaemia, and the serum potassium should be measured 2–4 weeks after starting treatment. The dose of the potassium-sparing drug may then need to be adjusted. The majority of patients have none of the special features listed in Table 3.5, and can be treated safely with the thiazide or loop diuretic alone. The average patient on an average dose of frusemide (40–80 mg daily) will have a serum potassium concentration of about 4.0–4.2 mmol/l – and this clearly needs no action. However, a small minority of patients do become markedly hypokalaemic, and the serum potassium should be measured 2–4 weeks after starting treatment. If it has fallen below 3.0 mmol/l a potassium-sparing drug should be added, and the dose should then be adjusted as required. When it is established that the serum potassium is within the acceptable range there is no need for further routine measurements. Of course it may need to be re-measured if circumstances change, for example after an increase in diuretic dosage or during an intercurrent illness.

Potassium-sparing diuretics. Spironolactone is more potent in preventing or correcting diuretic-induced hypokalaemia than amiloride or triamterene at the doses recommended by the manufacturers. Doses higher than 100 mg daily often cause gynaecomastia and should be avoided. Potassium-sparing drugs can cause life-threatening hyperkalaemia, and should not be used, in the following circumstances:

- when renal impairment is present (serum creatinine more than >130 μmol/l);
- with potassium supplements;
- with angiotensin converting enzyme (ACE) inhibitors, e.g. captopril, enalapril.

It follows that renal function *must* be measured before prescribing a potassium-sparing drug, even in the combined tablet forms listed in Table 3.6.

Combined diuretic therapy – when heart failure persists, despite moderate doses of a loop diuretic and vasodilator therapy (as will be discussed below), the dose of the loop diuretic can be increased as required. If dose increments give no further response secondary hyperaldosteronism may have developed, and the aldosterone antagonist spironolactone should be added to treatment (observing the contraindications mentioned above). This often enhances the

Table 3.6 Combined preparations containing a potassium-sparing drug. Measurement of renal function before prescribing is mandatory. The fixed dose of potassium-sparing drug may not prevent hypokalaemia

Containing amiloride	Containing spironolactone	Containing triamterene
Frumil	Aldactide	Dyazide
Moducren	Lasilactone	Dytide
Moduretic	Spiroprop	Frusene
Normetic		Kalspare
Synuretic		Triamco
Kalten		

response to the loop diuretic. If the response remains inadequate a large diuresis can often be attained by adding a thiazide diuretic to the regimen. One is then blocking three major sites of renal tubular sodium reabsorption – the ascending loop of Henle (loop diuretic), the cortical diluting segment (thiazide), and the site of Na : K exchange (spironolactone). This manoeuvre can lead to severe electrolyte disturbance, renal impairment and hypovolaemia, and should be undertaken only under the closest supervision and with very frequent biochemical monitoring. When this fails the prognosis is grim. A diuresis may sometimes be achieved by giving the loop diuretic intravenously, intermittently or by constant infusion, or by adding aminophylline to the treatment regimen.

Monitoring the response to treatment – the patient's subjective response, for example improvement in fatigue and dyspnoea, is obviously important, but unfortunately these symptoms are greatly influenced by factors quite unrelated to the heart failure, factors such as depression, family difficulties, etc. it is useful to have some objective measure of response. In chronic right heart failure *regular weighing is the simplest and most accurate measure of response*. One should aim for weight loss of 0.5 kg (1 lb) per day. Weight loss exceeding 1 kg per day is too fast, and suggests excessive diuresis which may cause severe electrolyte disturbance, hypovolaemia and renal failure. In chronic left heart failure the response can be assessed by auscultating the lung bases, observing whether the patient can lie flat comfortably, and by repeating the chest X-ray if pleural transudates were present initially. A simple walking test can also be useful, measuring for example the distance the patient can walk in a set time, or the time taken to walk a fixed distance.

In the initial phases of treatment, and particularly when diuretics are being used at high dosage or in combination, it is necessary to watch for hypokalaemia, hyponatraemia and a rising serum creatinine concentration. When the patient's condition and treatment are stable further routine checks are generally unnecessary, with the exception of an annual urine test for glycosuria.

When should vasodilators be added?

This question cannot be answered with any certainty at present. The best evidence comes from one very small study of patients with heart failure which was incompletely controlled by frusemide 40 mg daily[4]. The effects of increasing the dose of frusemide to 120 mg daily, or of adding the ACE inhibitor captopril 150 mg daily to frusemide 40 mg daily, were compared. The increased dose of frusemide proved the more effective of the two regimens as regards improvement of symptoms and increase in exercise tolerance. This suggests that vasodilators should be added only when moderately high doses of diuretic fail to control the heart failure. On the limited evidence available one should probably introduce vasodilators in the following circumstances:

- when there is a progressive rise in serum creatinine;
- serum sodium falls below 130 mmol/l;
- salt and water depletion develops, as evidenced by severe thirst with increasing doses of frusemide;
- there is no response to increasing doses of frusemide;
- heart failure remains uncontrolled by frusemide 250 mg daily.

These criteria may well need to be altered as new evidence becomes available.

Vasodilator treatment

General – the aim of vasodilator therapy is to reduce the afterload by arteriolar dilatation, reduce the preload by venodilation, and thus increase the contractility and reduce the work of the heart (Figure 3.1). It is conventional at this stage to list every vasodilator which exists, but only two forms of treatment which produce 'balanced' vasodilatation of both arterioles and veins are of proven value. The first is the use of an ACE inhibitor alone, i.e. enalapril or captopril, and the second the use of hydralazine plus isosorbide dinitrate in combination. Prazosin should no longer be used in heart failure, as its efficacy is not sustained and it does not improve the prognosis[1].

ACE inhibitors – a study published recently, the Consensus Trial[2], threatens to revolutionize the management of heart failure. In this study patients with severe heart failure (i.e. symptoms at rest) who were already on treatment with diuretics at high dosage, digoxin, and in some cases vasodilators, were randomly allocated to receive additional treatment with the ACE inhibitor enalapril, or with placebo. Enalapril treatment reduced the mortality after 6 months from 44% (placebo) to 25%. Enalapril also improved the patient's symptoms, reduced the heart size, and reduced the need for other anti-failure drugs. These striking benefits were obtained at the cost of hypotension and a decline in renal function in some patients, but these proved to be relatively minor problems. It is thus clear that enalapril has a major impact upon the morbidity and mortality of patients with severe heart failure, even when they are already treated with digoxin and high doses of diuretic. It should be emphasized that we do not know what relevance these observations have to patients with *mild* heart failure.

Enalapril or captopril? Captopril is also effective in relieving the symptoms of heart failure,[5] and it may cause less hypotension and renal impairment than enalapril because of its shorter duration of action[6]. On the other hand, it is more likely than enalapril to cause skin rashes and taste disturbance. There seems little to choose

MANAGEMENT OF HEART FAILURE

between the two drugs, but one should probably prefer enalapril at present in view of the results of the Consensus Trial.

Use of ACE inhibitors. The side-effects of ACE inhibitors are shown in Table 3.7. Profound hypotension after the first dose is by far the most important problem in practice, and is particularly likely to occur in patients taking high doses of diuretics and those with renal impairment or hyponatraemia. The initial dose has to be low (enalapril 2.5 mg, captopril 6.25 mg), must be taken when recumbent, and the patient has to be observed closely for at least 4 hours afterwards. Starting an ACE inhibitor in heart failure is not for the faint-hearted – it is best done in hospital. The other side-effect of note is persistent dry cough. Perhaps understandably the relation of this symptom to drug therapy is often overlooked, and patients may be subjected to much inappropriate treatment and extensive investigation before the penny drops.

Table 3.7 Side-effects of the angiotensin converting enzyme (ACE) inhibitors captopril and enalapril

First-dose hypotension	particularly in those taking diuretics, elderly and those with hyponatraemia or renal failure
Renal failure	particularly in patients with renovascular disease, or pre-existing renal failure
Hyperkalaemia	avoid potassium supplements and potassium-sparing drugs
Persistent cough	often misdiagnosed
Taste disturbance	more common with captopril
Skin rashes	more common with captopril
Angioedema	
Nasal congestion	reported only recently
Deafness	
Agranulocytosis	has occurred during captopril treatment, but can be avoided by following the manufacturers recommendations as regards dosage; dose adjustment in renal failure, drug interactions, and contraindications

Hydralazine plus isosorbide dinitrate – this regimen was compared to placebo in another 'landmark' study[1]. Patients with moderate heart failure, who were already on diuretics and digoxin, were treated either with the combined vasodilator regimen or placebo in addition to their standard anti-failure treatment. Over 2 years hydralazine plus isosorbide dinitrate reduced the mortality by one quarter, from 34% to 26%. This difference just reached statistical significance, and the outcome somewhat less clear-cut than that in the Consensus Trial. It should also be noted that the dose of hydralazine used, 300 mg daily, is likely to cause a lupus-like syndrome in an unacceptably high proportion of patients.

Which vasodilator regimen – On the evidence available an ACE inhibitor should probably be preferred to the hydralazine plus isosorbide dinitrate combination. ACE inhibitors are simpler to use, may be better tolerated, may be safer in the long-term, and may be more effective in reducing mortality.

Digoxin

Role in therapy – Some will be surprised that digoxin appears at this late stage in a review of the treatment of heart failure. It should be emphasized that it remains the cornerstone of treatment when heart failure is caused or accompanied by atrial fibrillation with a rapid ventricular rate. However, it has a very limited role in the management of patients in sinus rhythm – it is not very effective, it is difficult to use, and it is more likely to cause toxicity in such patients. It does have a measurable positive inotropic effect in the short term, and this may persist in some patients with more severe failure. Its use should not be abandoned entirely in patients with sinus rhythm, but it is best reserved for those whose failure remains uncontrolled by diuretic plus vasodilator treatment. It should be discontinued if improvement is not observed.

Prescribing digoxin – an oral dose is required only when there is an element of urgency, and it is doubtful whether the drug ever needs to be given intravenously. It is generally adequate, and certainly safer to start treatment with the predicted maintenance dose. The full effect will then develop over 7–14 days. The appropriate main-

Table 3.8 Average maintenance dose of digoxin in relation to renal function and age

Serum creatinine	Daily dose
< 150 μmol/l	250 μg
150–300 μmol/l	125 μg
> 300 μmol/l	62.5 μg
Age > 70 years:	62.5–125 μg daily

These doses are in general conservative, and the dose may need to be increased according to the response or as guided by measurement of the serum digoxin concentration

Table 3.9 Symptoms of digoxin toxicity. Note that arrhythmias may occur without any warning in the form of subjective symptoms

anorexia	visual disturbance
nausea	confusion
vomiting	ectopic beats
diarrhoea	arrhythmia (almost any)
abdominal pain	bradycardia
fatigue	heart block

tenance dose is determined largely by renal function and age, and guidelines are given in Table 3.8. It is stressed that these doses are only approximations. They will prove inadequate in some patients, and will cause toxicity in others, so that careful supervision is still needed. The response to digoxin treatment can be assessed relatively easily in patients with atrial fibrillation and a fast ventricular response. The dose is adjusted to attain a ventricular rate at rest of 60–80 beats per minute, measured by auscultation at the apex, while taking care to avoid symptoms and signs of digoxin toxicity (Table 3.9). The patient should be warned clearly about the symptoms which suggest toxicity, and should be advised to discontinue the drug and seek advice immediately if they occur. Patients in atrial fibrillation can usually be treated adequately without measuring serum digoxin levels, but knowledge of the serum digoxin concentration is helpful when the response to average doses is inadequate;

HEART FAILURE

Table 3.10 Summary of the treatment of chronic heart failure

Step 1	*Ensure* diagnosis correct	
Step 2	*Seek and treat* any correctable cause or precipitant (Table 2.1)	digoxin if atrial fibrillation with rapid ventricular rate
Step 3	*Diuretics:* Thiazide ↓ Loop diuretic (titrate dose) ↓ add spironolactone ↓ add thiazide	*Monitor:* body weight renal function electrolytes
Step 4	*Vasodilators* – add to diuretic treatment if: – renal function declines – hyponatraemia – hypotension, thirst, weakness – failure uncontrolled by frusemide 250 mg daily	
	enalapril 2.5 mg daily ↓ up to 40 mg daily	alternatives: captopril, or hydralazine plus isosorbide dinitrate
Step 5	Add *digoxin*, titrate dose according to serum digoxin concentration. Stop if there is no response	
Step 6	*Consider:* – non-compliance – interacting drugs – malabsorption of diuretics → i.v. frusemide – oral aminophylline	

when there is doubt about compliance; and when there is doubt whether symptoms such as anorexia or nausea indicate toxicity. If digoxin is used in patients in sinus rhythm measurements of the serum concentration are indispensable, as there are no useful clinical end-points against which the dose can be titrated. The dose should be adjusted to bring the serum digoxin concentration to the upper part of the therapeutic range (0.8–2.0 mg/ml).

Other inotropic drugs

Dopamine and dobutamine are widely used, by intravenous infusion, in patients with cardiogenic shock, but it is doubtful whether they alter the grim prognosis of this condition. The search for orally-active inotropic agents which would prove safe and effective for long-term use has to date proved fruitless, and there is some concern that such drugs might actually worsen the prognosis of heart failure.

Summary

The main points in the management of chronic heart failure are drawn together in Table 3.10.

ACUTE LEFT VENTRICULAR FAILURE

It is a relief to report that the management of acute left ventricular failure has not changed greatly in recent years – at least as it relates to general practice. A plan of management appropriate for treatment at home is outlined in Table 3.11. There are a few points of interest.

Frusemide – It is now clear that frusemide has a short-lived but important venodilator action when it is given intravenously. The symptoms of left ventricular failure are improved by 'unloading' the heart even before the diuresis begins.

Diamorphine – should be given intravenously, as absorption is inconsistent and slow after intramuscular injection. The dose should be reduced in the elderly, and it should be avoided altogether in patients with significant obstructive airways disease. It can cause

HEART FAILURE

Table 3.11 Management of acute left ventricular failure

Step 1	Frusemide 20–80 mg i.v. plus Diamorphine 2.5–5 mg i.v.	avoid diamorphine in those with chronic airways disease low dose for the elderly (naloxone must be to hand)
Step 2	Aminophylline 250 mg i.v.	inject very slowly. Be certain that patient is not already already taking a theophyllinate
Step 3	Glyceryl trinitrate 0.3–1.2 mg sublingually (according to tolerance)	
Step 4	Nifedipine 10–20 mg by buccal absorption	patient should bite capsule and hold juice in mouth

serious respiratory depression, and intravenous naloxone (0.1–0.2 mg) must be readily available whenever it is used.

Aminophylline – Intravenous aminophylline can cause serious arrhythmias or convulsions, and this is a particular risk in patients who are already taking a theophylline derivative orally. Aminophylline should be used only if left ventricular failure does not respond to frusemide and diamorphine, and only if one can be *certain* that the patient is not already taking an oral theophylline preparation.

Vasodilators – Parenteral vasodilator treatment is not a feasible proposition in the patient's home, but effective therapy can be improvised when necessary by using sublingual glyceryl trinitrate (venodilator) and nifedipine in capsule form (arteriolar dilator).

TERMINAL HEART FAILURE

Cardiac transplantation should be given some thought when all else fails. In general it may be considered in patients aged less than 60 years who have a very limited prognosis because of heart failure, and who are fit in other respects. The 5-year survival is of the order of 65% after transplantation, and the quality of life attained is very acceptable.

It is important to recognize the point in the progression of heart failure when death becomes inevitable. Further attempts to 'control' the failure will then merely cause discomfort with no prospect of real benefit to the patient. Death from terminal left ventricular failure is as unpleasant as any, and the principles of terminal care which come readily to mind when treating patients with malignancy often seem to be overlooked in these patients. Appropriate use of adequate doses of diamorphine are often a blessing in this situation.

REFERENCES

1. Cohn, J.N., Archibald, D.G., Ziesche, S., Franciosa, J.A., Harston, W.E., Tristani, F.E., Dunkman, W.B., Jacobs, W., Francis, G.S., Flohr, K.H., Goldman, H.S., Hughes, V.C. and Baker, B (1986). Effect of vasodilator therapy on mortality in chronic congestive heart failure. Results of a Veterans Administration Cooperative Study. *N. Engl. J. Med.*, 314, 1547–52
2. The Consensus Trial Study Group. (1987). Effects of enalapril on mortality in severe congestive heart failure. Results of the Cooperative North Scandinavian enalapril survival study (Consensus). *N. Engl. J. Med.*, 316, 1429–35
3. Davidson, C. (1985). Diuretic-induced hypokalaemia: factors influencing prevalence. In: *Diuretics in Heart Failure. Royal Society of Medicine International Congress and Symposium Series*, 83, 51–7
4. Cowley, A.J., Stainer, K., Wynne, R.D., Rowley, J.M. and Hampton, J.R. (1986). Symptomatic assessment of patients with heart failure: double-blind comparison of increasing doses of diuretics and captopril in moderate heart failure. *Lancet*, 2, 770–2
5. Bayliss, J., Norell, M.S., Canepa–Anson, R., Reid, C., Poole-Wilson, P. and Sutton, G. (1985). Clinical importance of the renin-angiotensin system in chronic heart failure; double-blind comparison of captopril and prazosin. *Br. Med. J.*, 290, 1861–5
6. Packer, M., Lee, W.H., Yushak, M. and Medina, N. (1986). Comparison of captopril and enalapril in patients with severe chronic heart failure. *N. Engl. J. Med.*, 315, 847–53

4 Surgical management of heart disease

N.J. Odom and C.G.A. McGregor

INTRODUCTION

Cardiac surgery has evolved since the 1950s, from a high risk and experimental undertaking, to providing safe, predictable and effective therapy for many cardiac conditions.

The principal factors contributing to this progress include the development of safe cardiopulmonary bypass, better surgical techniques, improved postoperative monitoring and intensive care, and the application of hypothermic cardioplegia allowing surgery on the motionless empty heart which is protected from ischaemic injury during the period of absent coronary blood flow.

Alongside the advances in surgical techniques, there have been equally important advances in diagnostic cardiology, including cardiac catheterization and echocardiography. Further notable developments include echo Doppler, which can measure the velocity of blood flow across valves and other orifices allowing pressure gradients to be measured non-invasively, and colour Doppler echo by which blood flow can be displayed visually enabling non-invasive diagnosis of a wide variety of conditions, such as septal defects and valvular regurgitation. Similarly, intervention cardiology has progressed from earlier techniques of balloon septostomy to those of valvotomy, angioplasty and vessel occlusion without the need of open surgical operation.

Over the past 10–20 years, there have been several long-term studies carried out on the natural history of cardiac disease, both with and without surgical treatment. This has enabled the long-term benefits of surgical therapy to be more fully understood. Nowadays, the risks and benefits of a particular operation can be based on more sound scientific information, rather than on anecdotal experience. Of particular importance in this regard are the long-term results of prosthetic valve replacement, and the impact of coronary artery surgery on late survival.

The aim of this chapter is to review current surgical treatment for ischaemic, valvular and terminal myocardial disease including patient selection, optimal timing of surgery and early and long-term results.

ISCHAEMIC HEART DISEASE

Ischaemic heart disease results from atherosclerosis in the coronary arteries. It presents as sudden death, acute myocardial infarction or as angina pectoris. Coronary artery bypass grafting (CABG) for angina is the commonest cardiac surgery. Indications for coronary artery surgery include:

- chronic stable angina, unresponsive to medical treatment;
- unstable or 'crescendo' angina;
- acute coronary occlusion during catheterization or angioplasty; and
- for prognostic considerations.

The decision to refer a patient for consideration of coronary grafting is only made after investigation by a cardiologist, notably by coronary arteriography. A major consideration, therefore, is patient selection for coronary arteriography.

Clearly a patient who is unable to work because of chronic stable angina or whose angina is worsening in severity or frequency should be referred for investigation. We know now that in certain groups of patients, the risk of dying from myocardial infarction can be reduced by coronary grafting. The commonest mode of presentation of ischaemic heart disease is sudden death, and so the potential value of treatment for prognostic considerations becomes clear.

Routine investigation of a patient presenting with angina consists of chest radiography, electrocardiography (ECG) and measurement of fasting lipid levels. It is necessary to exclude concomitant aortic valve disease, coarctation of the aorta, hypertension, hyperthyroidism and anaemia. The next phase of investigation is an exercise ECG to reveal whether or not large areas of myocardium become ischaemic on exercise. This would indicate significant proximal stenosis of one or more major coronary arteries, which may be of prognostic significance.

Definitive investigation is, of course, by selective coronary arteriography, to demonstrate the anatomical features of the disease. Left ventriculography will show how well the left ventricle is functioning, and will outline the position of akinetic segments from previous infarcts. It is only after undertaking coronary arteriography that a decision can be made as to the feasibility, risk, extent and prognostic implications of any proposed surgery.

Coronary arteriography is indicated in any patient for whom surgical therapy is being considered, including patients with disabling chronic angina, those with worsening (crescendo) angina, and those in whom exercise ECG indicates a large area of myocardium under threat.

Once operative treatment has been decided upon, surgery should be carried out as soon as is practicable. The timing of surgery for chronic stable angina in the UK is, in practice, determined by the length of the surgical waiting list, rather than by medical considerations. As a result, many coronary artery grafts have to be performed on an urgent, or semi-urgent basis on patients in the medical wards or on the coronary care unit, who have angina uncontrolled by maximum medical therapy. Due to inadequate facilities for coronary surgery in the UK, there is a significant mortality on the waiting list for coronary artery bypass grafting.

The operation itself consists of the removal of the long saphenous vein from the calf and/or thigh, and grafting segments of vein

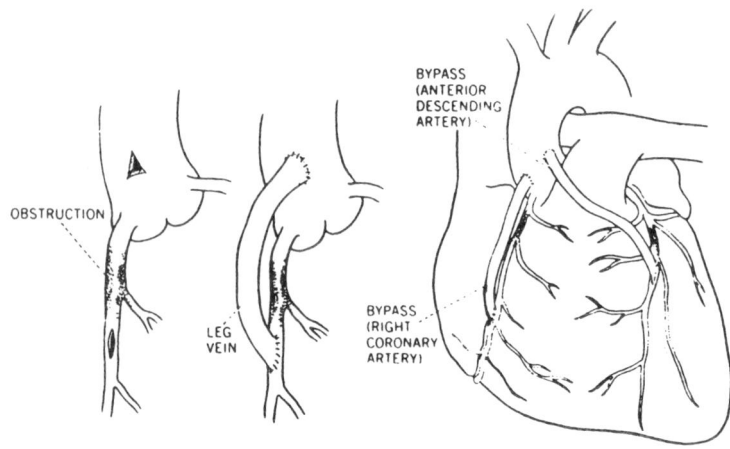

Figure 4.1 Coronary artery bypass grafting

end to side onto the diseased coronary arteries, distal to the obstructing lesions. (Figure 4.1) The proximal ends of the grafts are then joined to the side of the ascending aorta. Between one and seven grafts may be performed; the average number per patient is around three. Often, one length of vein is used to graft two or more coronary arteries, using side-to-side anastomoses – so-called 'jump' or 'sequential' grafts. The operation generally lasts for between 3 and 4 hours, and the patient is nursed on intensive care for about 24–48 hours. The patient is usually discharged home about a week after operation, and may return to work after 6–8 weeks. Heavy work, or lifting heavy objects, should be avoided for 10 weeks, until the sternotomy incision has fully healed.

The overall operative mortality for CABG[2] is about 3%. Uncomplicated cases should have a mortality of about 1%; patients with unstable angina or with poor ventricular function have a higher mortality. Most deaths result from myocardial infarction around the time of surgery usually due to inadequate myocardial preservation or suboptimal revascularization. In addition to the operative mortality, there is a risk of major morbidity, such as a cerebrovascular accident or significant infection, of around 3% each.

The symptomatic benefits of CABG are considerable. Nowadays, over 80% of patients are free from angina at 1 year following surgery. Of those patients who continue to suffer from angina, about half are significantly improved, and can be managed satisfactorily on medical treatment.

The major cause of early recurrent angina, (i.e. angina following CABG) is thrombosis of the vein grafts. This may occur early after operation due to technical complications, or if the flow of blood down the graft is too low to sustain patency, (i.e. poor 'run-off'). Late recurrent angina occurring months or years after surgery is due to the development of intimal hyperplasia in the vein grafts and/or progression of disease in the native coronary arteries. This process can be retarded by the use of anti-platelet drugs, and most patients undergoing CABG will receive aspirin and dipyridamole for up to a year after operation[3]. The rate of recurrence of angina beyond one year after surgery is approximately 2–4% per year[4]. Although it was clear that symptomatic improvement in angina was dramatic following CABG, it was not known for how long this improvement would last, or whether the incidence of myocardial infarction or death was altered.

As a result, the long-term benefits of coronary artery surgery have been studied in three major multicentre trials, namely the Veterans' Administration Cooperative Study and the Coronary Artery Surgery Study (CASS) in the United States, and the European Coronary Artery Surgery Study. In these trials, patients with moderate angina were prospectively randomized to receive medical or surgical treatment. Initially, no overall differences in survival were demonstrated between patients treated medically or surgically[5]. With longer follow-up, however, clear advantages of surgical treatment over medical treatment became apparent, both in terms of survival, and in reduction of the incidence of myocardial infarction[6]. In the European study, certain subgroups of patients were identified in whom surgery clearly reduced the risk of subsequent death from myocardial infarction[7].

For the purpose of description, the coronary vasculature can be divided into three major systems; the two major branches of the

HEART FAILURE

left coronary artery, the left anterior descending (LAD) and the circumflex, and the right coronary artery.

Most patients with disease affecting one or two systems will not be at major risk of death from myocardial infarction, and will not have an improved prognosis following surgery. There are, however, three patterns of disease that have been identified as carrying a significant risk of death, and in which surgical treatment will reduce this risk. These three patterns of disease that have been identified as carrying a significant risk of death, and in which surgical treatment will reduced this risk. These three patterns are as follows:

- 'triple vessel disease'; i.e. when all three major branches of the coronary tree are stenosed, associated with impaired left ventricular function;
- stenosis of the main stem of the left coronary artery; and
- proximal stenosis of the LAD i.e. before the major septal and diagonal branches.

Occlusion of such a stenosed segment is liable to result in a major infarct with a high mortality. As such, these patterns of disease are in themselves relative indications for surgical treatment on prognostic grounds, even in the presence of only mild angina.

The European study showed an improved survival for patients treated surgically who had triple vessel disease. The survival figures at 5 years in the surgically treated and medically treated groups were 91% and 73% respectively. Corresponding figures for proximal LAD disease were 90% in the surgical group and 79% in the medical group. (These figures do, of course, include the operative mortality in the surgical group.) It must be remembered that these figures represent patients with mild or moderate angina; patients with severe angina would have undergone surgical therapy in any case, and therefore, excluded from the trial.

Patients with rapidly worsening or 'crescendo' angina require urgent coronary arteriography as many will have severe proximal lesions. Also, patients who suffer a small infarct, but who continue to suffer from chest pain, should also be investigated, as often there is a major area of jeopardized myocardium which can be saved by timely revascularization.

SURGICAL MANAGEMENT OF HEART DISEASE

Surgery also has a role to play following myocardial infarction. Most cardiologists would agree that patients should undergo exercise ECG 4–6 weeks following their first infarct. If there are widespread ischaemic changes on exercise, then coronary angiography should be performed. If the patient has significant proximal stenoses of prognostic significance (as previously described), then surgery should be recommended to prevent further infarction. This will apply even if the patient has minimal or no symptoms of angina.

Acute coronary occlusion during cardiac catheterization or angioplasty is amenable to treatment by emergency CABG. Surgery has also been proposed for treatment of acute myocardial infarction; however, it requires to be performed in under 6 hours from the onset of symptoms in order to salvage a significant quantity of myocardium[8]. This approach has not gained widespread acceptance.

A more practical approach to the treatment of acute infarction is the immediate use of an intravenous thrombolytic agent, such as streptokinase, urokinase, or more recently, tissue plasminogen activator (TPA). This therapy is most appropriate for the younger patient, without a history of peptic ulcer disease or other bleeding disorders; such treatment if started as soon as possible after ECG confirmation of the diagnosis, may prevent major myocardial loss, especially in anteroseptal infarction. The patient should then be transferred to an invasive cardiology unit, where angiography and intracoronary thrombolysis with the same agent can be carried out[9]. If the left anterior descending coronary artery cannot be recannulized rapidly, then angioplasty (see below) should be performed. This aggressive approach to the management of a major coronary occlusion in an otherwise healthy patient may abort major infarction with significant mortality[10].

Patients with angina and impairment of left ventricular function from previous infarction are amenable to CABG. Poor ventricular function as a result of ischaemia may improve following revascularization, although infarcted areas, of course, will not recover. CABG can be performed with acceptable risks in the presence of angina even if the left ventricular ejection fraction is as low as 15%. CABG is unlikely to improve shortness of breath, but will often abolish or reduce angina.

The upper age limit for CABG is determined mainly by the degree of provision of services for heart surgery, rather than by age *per se*. Provided the patient is otherwise healthy, good results can be obtained in people in their seventies or older. However, such patients are unlikely to be investigated and operated on by units in the UK where people in their forties are having to wait several months for the investigation and surgical treatment of chronic stable angina.

There are two specific techniques for myocardial revascularization which deserve separate mention.

The internal mammary artery (IMA) is being increasingly used to bypass coronary arteries, instead of using segments of long saphenous vein. The artery is dissected off the posterior chest wall at the beginning of the operation, and detached at its lower end. The distal end is then anastomosed directly to the side of the coronary artery, usually the LAD. The advantage of using the IMA is that the long-term patency is superior to saphenous vein. Intimal hyperplasia does not occur, and long-term patency is greater than 95%[11].

Unfortunately, only one or two anastomoses can be constructed using the IMA, and it will not reach some vessels on the posterior and diaphragmatic surfaces of the heart. Nevertheless, it is the ideal conduit for lesions of the LAD artery, and is being increasingly used, either on its own, or in combination with vein grafts to other coronary branches as required.

The other technique is percutaneous transluminal coronary angioplasty (PTCA). This is performed by a radiologist or cardiologist in the cardiac catheterization laboratory. A small balloon is passed over a guide-wire under direct screening, so as to traverse a stenosed segment of coronary of artery. The balloon is then inflated, thereby dilating the stenosis.

The ideal lesion to treat by this method is one which is less than 3 months old, is concentric in shape, and which does not involve the origins of side branches. Patients with single vessel disease are better suited to angioplasty than those with multi-vessel disease.

The decision to perform angioplasty as opposed to surgery is made by the cardiologist, after seeing the coronary angiogram. There is a significant learning curve to be overcome with this technique; however, with increased experience, PTCA is being performed on a wider variety of patients, such as those with two or three vessel disease. After the learning curve is past, failure to relieve the stenosis will occur in about 23% of cases[12]. In addition, there is a small but significant risk of acute coronary occlusion, usually as a result of coronary dissection, occurring in up to 6% of cases[13]. For this reason, it is necessary to have a surgical team available so that emergency coronary grafting can be carried out if required.

The advantage of PTCA over CABG is the decreased cost and morbidity. The patient can be discharged home within 2 days, and can return to work thereafter. There is, however, a significant incidence of stenosis after PTCA, of approximately 34% after 5 months[14], but repeat PTCA is equally effective and so this is not necessarily as discouraging as it sounds[15]. The long-term results in the remaining patients appear encouraging, and PTCA may be applicable to up to 10 or 15% of patients requiring myocardial revascularization. It is unlikely to replace surgery, however, as the treatment of choice for patients with multi-vessel disease.

Coronary surgery and angioplasty are very effective therapy for angina, and will in some cases improve prognosis. These treatments are, however, only palliative, and will not themselves prevent the progression of atherosclerosis. For this reason, preventative measures, both in the population as a whole and following surgery are of paramount importance in the prevention of death from myocardial infarction. There is considerable room for improvement in the screening of blood lipid profiles and in the control of hypercholesterolaemia by diet; also in certain cases by appropriate medication, such as cholestyramine, nicotinic acid or lovastatin.

With a 2–4% incidence of recurrent angina beyond one year after CABG in addition to the 10–15% initial failure rate, it can be seen that after 10 years, nearly half the patients operated on will have recurrent angina. Repeat coronary surgery can be performed, albeit with an increased operative risk[2], but an operative mortality for repeat CABG of around 3% is achievable[16].

HEART FAILURE

Certain complications of acute myocardial infarction can also be treated surgically. These include ruptured interventricular septum, ruptured papillary muscle causing acute mitral regurgitation and left ventricular aneurysm. Patients with medically refractory ventricular tachyarrhythmias associated with coronary disease can be treated by concomitant electrophysiological mapping and endocardial resection.

In summary:

- prevention is better than cure; screening and control of risk factors, such as hypertension, hypercholesterolaemia and smoking are of great importance.
- the primary goal at every stage in the management of the patient with evolving coronary artery occlusion is limitation of infarct size.
- all patients with angina, or who are diagnosed as having coronary artery disease, should have an exercise ECG, in order to elucidate the possible presence of a major life-threatening coronary stenosis.
- increased availability of specialist cardiological services and facilities for more coronary artery surgery are required in the UK.

VALVULAR HEART DISEASE

The valves most commonly affected by acquired disease are the mitral and aortic valves. The tricuspid valve is usually only affected in the presence of severe mitral valve disease, endocarditis, and in rare conditions such as carcinoid disease and drug dependency.

Rheumatic heart disease remains the commonest indication for valve replacement in the UK. The incidence of rheumatic fever has decreased in recent decades. Effects of this change on valve replacement surgery is delayed as valve lesions occur late after the initial illness, but there are indications that the age range of patients having valve replacement for rheumatic disease is increasing in the UK. It does, however, occur in a younger age group in the immigrant communities, and remains a significant problem in Third World countries. Other causes of chronic aortic valve disease include senile aortic valve sclerosis and connective tissue disorders such as Marfan's syndrome. Causes of acute aortic valve regurgitation include endocarditis, aortic dissection and trauma. Acute mitral regurgitation can result from ruptured chordae or ruptured papillary muscle from ischaemic or degenerative disease, endocarditis or trauma. In most cases urgent valve replacement is necessary to control left ventricular failure.

Most chronic valve disease is slowly progressive. Adaptive changes occur in the myocardium and pulmonary vasculature, so that the onset of symptoms may occur only late in the disease process. The optimal timing of surgical intervention is often difficult and has changed considerably since the introduction of prosthetic valve replacement in the late 1950s. In those early days, valve replacement was a treatment of last resort for a patient with pre-terminal heart failure. Operative mortality was extremely high, and recovery was limited by pre-existing permanent myocardial damage. When the operative risk diminished to acceptably low levels and the long-term reliability of prosthetic valves became known, surgery became recommended earlier in the disease process.

There are three advantages in recommending earlier surgery:

- patients are fitter when operated,on, so operative risk is minimized;
- patients can be spared periods of increasing disability as their disease progresses; and
- myocardial damage can be prevented by the restoration of normal haemodynamics.

Surgery should be timed to occur at the point when the risks and morbidity of allowing the disease process to continue unchecked exceed the risks and morbidity of operative intervention[17].

Alongside the advances in surgical technique and prosthetic valve development, there have been advances in the methods used to diagnose and assess the severity of valvular lesions. Cardiac catheterization used to be the only reliable way to quantitate the degree of haemodynamic abnormality. Echocardiography has now developed to such an extent that a precise anatomical and haemodynamic assessment is possible using only non-invasive methods[18]. Gradients across stenosed valves can be quantified by measuring the velocity of blood flow using the Doppler echo, and regurgitation can be demonstrated by the same technique. Modern developments in this field include colour flow imaging, (which allows blood flow patterns to be displayed visually superimposed on the 2 D echo), and the transoesophageal echo, which gives a degree of resolution previously unobtainable.

The vast majority of patients with valvular disease can be adequately assessed using echocardiography, and when interpreted in the clinical context, a decision can be made as to the best timing of operation. Cardiac catheterization is often unnecessary in the assessment of valve disease alone. It is, however, required in many older patients before surgery in order to determine the presence of concomitant coronary artery disease. Most surgeons would accept that significant coronary stenoses should be grafted at the time of valve replacement or repair, but the evidence for this approach is equivocal.

The first operations performed for valvular heart disease were attempts to dilate stenosed valves, while the heart was still beating; so-called 'closed' heart surgery. These procedures are no longer performed, except for critical aortic or pulmonary stenosis in neonates, and in certain cases of mitral stenosis in adults. The operation of closed mitral valvotomy gives excellent results if the patients are properly selected, in terms of clinical and echocardiographic features. The techniques of closed valvotomy is ideally suited to patients with pure mitral stenosis, in sinus rhythm, with no history of embolic episodes, and no echocardiographic evidence of valve calcification or left atrial thrombus. Contraindications to closed valvotomy include significant mitral regurgitation, valve calcification, chordal shortening, or evidence of left atrial thrombus. Some surgeons would regard atrial fibrillation as a contraindication to closed valvotomy; however, there is evidence that patients in atrial fibrillation do not have a higher incidence of perioperative embolism[19]. If these rather stringent criteria are adhered to, excellent results can be obtained. However, a decreasing number of these operations are currently performed in the UK, as fewer patients meet the criteria, and eventually it will probably cease to be performed as in the US, especially if the non-operative technique of trans-septal balloon valvoplasty becomes established[20]. In developing countries, however, closed mitral valvotomy is a very commonly performed and effective operation. Rheumatic fever is a common disease, and a rapidly progressive form of mitral stenosis may occur, which is ideally treated by closed valvotomy.

The majority of operations for aortic and mitral valve disease involve valve replacement. There is no ideal artificial valve. Although prosthetic valves can restore comparatively normal haemodynamics, they all carry significant morbidity. All prosthetic valves are subject to endocarditis, early and late, and antibiotic prophylaxis is required for life for dental treatment and other situations where bacteraemia might occur such as skin infections, penetrating injuries or surgical procedures, e.g. cystoscopy.

Artificial valves may be divided broadly into two types: mechanical and biological (Figure 4.2). Early mechanical valves were made of metal and plastic. The Starr–Edwards valve, which is of a 'ball and cage' construction, was the first successful mechanical valve. Modern versions of this valve are still used today: it is extremely rugged and reliable, although it is haemodynamically less efficient than more recent designs. Several versions of the tilting disk valve have been popular, but some have now fallen into disrepute. The best known tilting disk valve is the Bjork–Shiley valve, which has a good track record[21,22]. Disk valves undergo mechanical failure very rarely, but if they do, they may fail suddenly, with catastrophic results. Causes of valve failure include wedging of the disk in the open or closed position; this may be caused by valve thrombosis, or by a suture or chordae tendinae wedging in the disk. Strut fractures and disk embolization have also occurred. Good long-term survival has been reported[21,22]. The latest design of Bjork–Shiley valve is made of pyrolite carbon, and has a non-welded construction, which appears to reduce the risk of strut fracture. The most modern designs of mechanical valve are the bi-leaflet valves, such as the St Jude and the Duramedic. These are also made of

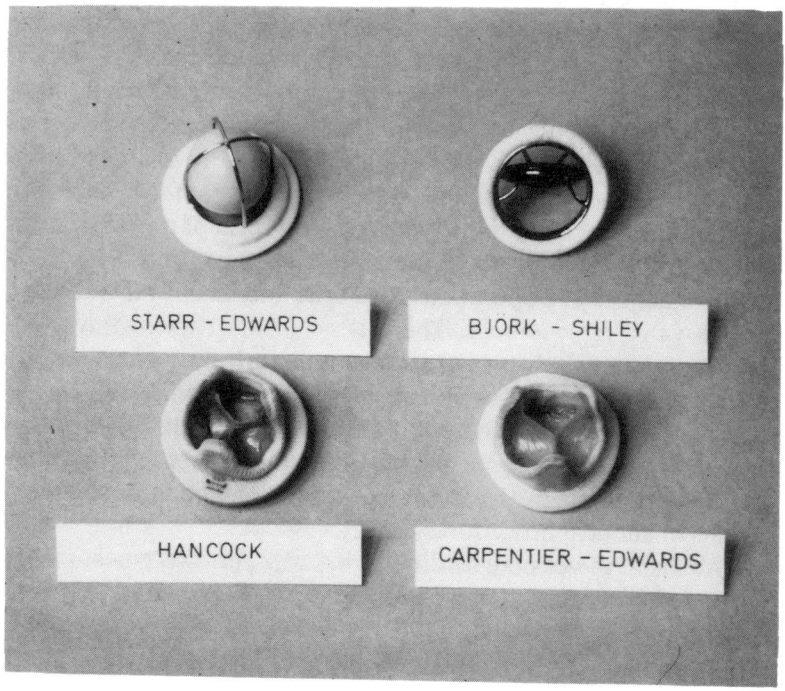

Figure 4.2 Mechanical and biological artificial valves

pyrolite carbon. The early experience with these prostheses is encouraging; they appear to be reliable, and have a relatively low propensity for causing thrombosis[23]. Recently, however, some Duramedic valves have undergone acute mechanical failure, due to dislodgement and embolization of one of the leaflets. In spite of the improvements in design over the years, all mechanical valves have the propensity to cause thrombosis and embolism, and all require lifelong anticoagulation. The only exception may be in children where some studies have suggested that antiplatelet therapy may be sufficient[24]. Anticoagulation itself carries a significant long-term risk of bleeding complications.

Biological valves are made from biological tissues. The commonest design is the glutaraldehyde-preserved porcine valve. Common makes include the Carpentier–Edwards, and Hancock valves[25,26]. Patients with these valves do not require long-term anticoagulation, unless there is another indication such as left atrial thrombosis or previous embolism. The disadvantage of these valves is that they undergo calcification and degeneration, resulting in valve failure. This tends to occur rapidly in children, and biological valves tend not to be used for aortic or mitral replacement in children or teenagers. In adults, most biological prostheses do very well for 7–10 years, after which there is a progressive attrition rate requiring repeat valve replacement. After 10 years, over 30% of valves will need to have been replaced. Failure usually occurs gradually, so that repeat surgery can be arranged before significant haemodynamic deterioration occurs. Recent evidence shows that valves made from bovine pericardium, such as the Ionescu–Shiley, have a more rapid attrition rate than porcine valves, and may fail suddenly when a cusp tears[27].

It is, of course, very important that patients with artificial valves are followed-up regularly, and that repeat surgery is carried out early after the onset of signs of valve failure. The usual sign of valve failure is the onset of regurgitation, as evidenced by a characteristic murmur. Echocardiography and Doppler can then be used to confirm the diagnosis, and quantify the haemodynamic disturbance. Failure may also result in the gradual onset of valve stenosis.

Repeat operation, although technically more difficult than first time operation, can be performed with an acceptably low mortality, provided surgery is carried out before the onset of severe heart failure. Although the necessity for repeat operation is a disadvantage when using a biological valve, the risk of repeat surgery is roughly balanced by the risks of anticoagulation for a mechanical valve, over the equivalent time span[28].

The general policy of many surgeons has been to use mechanical valves for younger patients and biological valves for older. Sometimes, a particular type of valve may be contraindicated; for example, mechanical valves should be avoided in people with a history of gastrointestinal haemorrhage or in women who wish to bear children. On the other hand, one would tend to avoid using a biological valve in a situation where repeat surgery would be particularly hazardous. If a biological valve is required for aortic valve replacement in a young person, probably the very best option would be a fresh homograft valve, removed from a cadaver, or from a heart removed from a heart transplant recipient. Unfortunately, these valves are in short supply, and only a few surgeons use them[29]. Beyond these broad guidelines, however, the choice of valve remains mainly one of personal preference on the part of the patient and surgeon. The operative mortality for valve replacement is approximately 3% for aortic, and 5% for mitral valve replacement.

A significant advance in recent years has been the development of techniques of mitral valve repair, originated by McGoon[30] and popularized by Carpentier[31]. These procedures can be performed only in selected patients with specific valvular defects amenable to correction. Valve repair is particularly applicable to the mitral and tricuspid valves. Mitral stenosis can be corrected by open commissurotomy in patients in whom closed valvotomy is contraindicated for whatever reason. Regurgitation due to annular dilatation can be corrected by annuloplasty, and certain other defects such as mitral cusp prolapse can be corrected by plicating or resecting part of the valve leaflet, or shortening the chordae tendinae. Studies comparing the long-term results of these procedures with the results of valve replacement show conflicting results[32–34] largely reflecting different selection criteria: valve repair will only give good long-term results if performed on valves which are not too severely damaged.

Pre-operative assessment of the patient by echocardiography will enable conservative operations to be planned carefully. The final decision as to whether repair is feasible, and as to the exact type of repair, can only be made at the time of surgery. The advantage of these conservative procedures is significant as haemodynamic abnormalities can be corrected with a lower morbidity and mortality than valve replacement. A more aggressive policy of echocardiographic assessment of patients with mild symptoms will allow more of these procedures to be performed, thereby preventing the onset of myocardial deterioration, and delaying the need for valve replacement.

SURGICAL MANAGEMENT OF HEART DISEASE

Conservative repair of the aortic valve has not achieved the same level of success as for the mitral. Patients in their seventies with calcific stenosis of a tricuspid aortic valve who are otherwise fit, may well be amenable to treatment by aortic valve decalcification. Gratifying long-term results will only be achieved if the valve is anatomically normal, i.e. with three cusps[35]. Devices such as the ultrasound probe can be used to facilitate this procedure. Aortic valve decalcification is becoming increasingly used in the USA and will no doubt become used in Britain, as a number of older people undergoing heart surgery increases. Anatomically normal valves, however, do not calcify until late in life; patients with calcific aortic stenosis presenting in their forties and fifties usually have bicuspid or otherwise abnormal valves which are not amenable to decalcification.

The indications for surgery in each of the different valve lesions will now be reviewed.

Mitral stenosis

Mitral stenosis causes an increased pressure in the pulmonary veins, and restricts the flow of blood into the left ventricle. Symptoms include diminished exercise tolerance and shortness of breath. Prolonged pulmonary venous hypertension leads to a rise in pulmonary vascular resistance; this further increases the pulmonary artery pressure, and may result in right ventricular failure.

The major indication for surgical intervention is symptomatic disability. Surgery should be performed before the onset of reduced cardiac output and right ventricular failure. The raised pulmonary vascular resistance increases the operative risk and may take up to 3 months to recover after operation.

Symptomatic deterioration in mitral stenosis frequently occurs with the onset of atrial fibrillation. The possibility of surgical intervention should be looked into at this time, especially if echocardiography indicates that closed valvotomy, or open repair may be feasible. Under these circumstances, most patients can be restored to sinus rhythm after operation, with a significant reduction in the long-term risk of thromboembolic complications.

Aortic stenosis

A pressure gradient across a stenosed aortic valve results in a 'compensatory' left ventricular hypertrophy. The onset of symptoms is an indication that the left ventricle is under considerable strain, and is of sinister prognostic significance. Symptoms may consist of angina, or effort syncope, In either case, surgery should be performed forthwith, as such a patient is at risk of sudden death. An alternative mode of presentation is left ventricular failure. In either case, symptoms occur only after considerable left ventricular strain has occurred. The pressure gradient of more than 50 mmHg across the aortic valve as measured by Doppler echo or direct cardiac catheterization is an indication for operation. In the presence of severe left ventricular dysfunction, however, the heart may be incapable of generating a high pressure gradient. Under these circumstances, a low pressure gradient should not lull one into a false sense of security, but valve replacement should be performed to prevent worsening left ventricular failure.

Mitral regurgitation

The indications for surgery for valvular regurgitation are far less well defined than for stenosis[17]. This applies both to mitral and aortic regurgitation. Both conditions result in an increased volume load to the left ventricle. Generally, an increased volume load is relatively well tolerated, and heart failure occurs late in the disease process. Many patients with moderate degrees of regurgitation may remain in a stable asymptomatic state for several years. Also, quantification of the degree of regurgitation is difficult. Nowadays, however, the echo Doppler allows a good assessment to be made of the degree of regurgitation, both in aortic and mitral valve disease.

Symptomatic deterioration occurs late in chronic mitral regurgitation. Valve replacement performed at this time can carry a high mortality as the left ventricle is suddenly faced with a competent valve, and has to eject against higher compensatory myocardial changes which is unable to cope with the sudden increase in outflow resistance[36]. Patients often require vasodilator therapy post-operatively to reduce the left ventricular afterload. Late in the disease process the patient's overall condition may not be improved by valve replacement as myocardial injury occurring as a result of chronic volume overload may fail to reverse.

For these reasons, surgery should be recommended earlier in the evolution of mitral regurgitation so that myopathic changes can be prevented and a good result obtained. The exact timing of intervention is a matter of fine judgement especially in a patient who has little or no symptoms.

Aortic regurgitation

Much that has been said about mitral regurgitation is also true of aortic regurgitation. However, replacement of the aortic valve will not result in an increased afterload as compared to before operation. It will, however, reduce the diastolic filling of the heart.

Nonetheless, it remains true that the adaptive changes in the myocardium to the increased volume load before surgery may be, to a large extent, irreversible. Therefore, it is important to operate before significant left ventricular dilatation occurs. Again, the timing of this decision may be difficult in a patient who is relatively asymptomatic[37]. As a rough guide, when the left ventricular systolic diameter reaches 5.5 cm, operation should be considered[38]. It is all too easy to defer operating on an apparently well patient. Delayed surgery may result in permanent myocardial damage with a resultant high operative risk.

In summary:
- symptoms are often a poor guide to the severity of cardiac valvular disease: echocardiography should be undertaken on

all patients with valvular disease to confirm the diagnosis, to quantify the haemodynamic abnormality, and to assess ventricular function;
- surgery should be carried out before severe ventricular damage has occurred. This is best achieved by regular patient review with echocardiography as required;
- all patients with prosthetic valves must take precautions to prevent bacterial endocarditis;
- all patients with mechanical valves will require close anticoagulant control for life;
- all patients with biological valves must be assessed periodically. The onset of a new murmur, or any change in the character of the prosthetic heart sounds or increase in heart size on chest X-ray is an indication for urgent investigation; and
- any sudden deterioration in the cardiac condition of a patient with a mechanical valve in place should be urgently investigated and considered secondary to valve malfunction until proven otherwise.

TERMINAL MYOCARDIAL DISEASE

Terminal myocardial disease is the end result of a number of different disease processes including cardiomyopathy and end-stage ischaemic disease. Medical treatment with diuretics and vasodilators will improve many of the symptoms of myocardial failure, but there is a limit to what can be achieve medically, and prognosis remains poor. The advent of cardiac transplantation offers the hope of prolonged survival with a relatively normal life-style, for selected patients with terminal heart failure. This should radically alter the approach that one takes to the assessment and subsequent management of such a patient.

The first human heart transplant was performed by Barnard in 1967[39]. Although there was a rash of cardiac transplants performed in the following year, survival was poor, and the procedure was largely abandoned. During the 1970's further developments took place, notably at Stanford University, and by 1979 the results were sufficiently promising to stimulate the reintroduction of heart transplantation in other centres.

Particularly important factors in achieving improved results have been stricter selection criteria for recipients and donors; the development of the endomyocardial biopsy technique for the diagnosis of rejection and the introduction of cyclosporin[40,41]. In addition, techniques of myocardial preservation, including cold cardioplegia, enable donor hearts to be retrieved from distant sites, without having to transport the body of the donor. This is now standard practice and greatly simplifies the logistics of obtaining donor organs.

Since 1980 the number of heart transplants in the UK and world-wide has increased each year. In 1987, over 200 heart transplants were performed in the four government funded centres at Papworth, Harefield, Newcastle and Manchester. The recent Brunel report indicated that potentially between 500 and 900 patients per year in Britain could benefit from cardiac transplantation[42]. At present, the major limiting factor is the provision of facilities and resources, but as the numbers expand, the ultimate limiting factor will be the availability of suitable donors.

The results of transplantation have continued to improve. Nowadays, heart transplantation should be regarded as a routine form of therapy for selected patients. The latest patient survival figures from Standford University are 83% at 1 year, and 60% at 5 years[43].

The indication for heart transplantation is terminal heart disease not amenable to conventional therapy. Life expectancy without transplantation would be in the order of months to a year or two. Most patients will be in NYHA class III or IV; however, certain patients with cardiomyopathy may have a very poor prognosis, in spite of appearing to be relatively well. Poor prognostic features in cardiomyopathy include an ejection fraction below 20%, or the presence of ventricular tachyarrhythmias[44]. Approximately half the suitable recipients for heart transplantation suffer from dilated cardiomyopathy; and the remainder from end-stage ischaemic heart disease. Other rarer conditions amenable to heart transplantation include end-stage valvular disease with myocardial failure, cardiac tumours and myocarditis.

Major contraindications to heart transplantation include active infections, poor renal or hepatic function, increased pulmonary vascular resistance, recent pulmonary infarction and severe psycho-social instability including non-compliance and drug abuse. Insulin-dependent diabetes was, until recently, an absolute contraindication, but now the requirement for the use of steroids for immunosuppression has been dramatically reduced so that stable diabetics can be successfully transplanted. Diabetes does, however, remain a relative contraindication.

The upper age limit for heart transplantation is around 55 years. This is mainly dictated by the availability of donors and resources rather than by any purely medical considerations. Biological rather than chronological age is important, and otherwise healthy patients over the age of 60 have been successfully transplanted.

The lower age limit has not been defined. The youngest transplant in Britain was performed at the age of 4 months. Neonates with complex congenital heart disease have been successfully transplanted in California, but this has not so far been achieved in Britain. Cardiac transplantation in the treatment of congenital heart disease will become increasingly common.

Assessment of potential recipients

Potential recipients are admitted to the hospital for an assessment before a final decision regarding transplantation can be made. At this time, a detailed history is taken and physical examination performed, with particular reference to any potential infective problems. Measurement of renal function is performed: in general, patients with a creatinine clearance of less than 30 ml/min will develop significant renal insufficiency following transplantation, and would not normally be accepted. Cardiac catheterization for measurement of pulmonary vascular resistance (PVR) is carried out: a PVR of greater than six Wood unit contraindicates orthotopic transplantation, although the exact upper limit is difficult to define, and may vary between patients. The serum of a potential cardiac recipient is tested for the presence of preformed antibodies against a panel of blood donor lymphocytes. If any of these tests are positive, then a direct crossmatch will be required before proceeding when a donor becomes available; otherwise, direct crossmatching is performed retrospectively. Arrangements are made for communicating with and transporting the patient when a donor becomes available. Acutely ill patients (such as those with myocarditis), may need to remain in hospital on medical therapy, and given priority when a suitable donor becomes available.

The waiting period is a time of considerable stress and uncertainty for patients. On the one hand is the knowledge that their condition may deteriorate, and that nearly one-third of patients accepted for transplantation die before a suitable donor heart can be found. On the other hand, there is a prospect of regaining health, albeit after major surgery and an uncertain recovery period. Some patients may experience guilt or anxiety over the knowledge that their lives can only be saved as the result of a tragic loss on the part of the donor family.

Donors

Cardiac donors must be diagnosed as brain dead according to the criteria laid down by the Royal Colleges, and be in a stable haemodynamic condition[45]. Donors over the age of 40 are not usually suitable for cardiac donation. Potential donors should not have suffered any prolonged period of hypotension, and should not require heavy inotropic support. Frequently, potential cardiac donors become hypovolaemic as a result of diabetes insipidus, or deliberate dehydration for treatment of cerebral injury. Rehydration will usually enable the inotropic support to be reduced or discontinued. The donor operation is arranged in conjunction with other donor teams who will be harvesting other organs. Donor and recipient operations are co-ordinated, so that the transport time and period of cardiac ischaemia is kept to a minimum.

Postoperative course

After operation, the recipient will remain in intensive care for a number of days. The recovery period is similar to that for conventional heart surgery, but precautions must be taken to avoid infection (such as reverse barrier nursing), and a close watch kept for evidence of rejection. Some patients may require temporary cardiac pacing, and a smaller number may require the insertion of a permanent cardiac pacemaker in order to prevent life-threatening bradycardias. The patient may be discharged home as early as 2 weeks after operation, if there are no complications. More than two-thirds of patients, however, have one or more episodes of rejection and/or infection during the first month after surgery, and this will, or course, delay discharge. Patients are required to remain near the hospital for 6 weeks, and to be followed-up closely for this period.

Cardiac biopsies are performed weekly for 6 weeks, and at other times if rejection is suspected. After 6 weeks, the frequency of biopsies and other follow-up visits is gradually reduced. Rejection is treated using a short, high-dose course of steroids.

After discharge, patients need to keep a close record of their drug protocol, their temperature and their weight. They will be on several medications; usually cyclosporin, azathioprine and steroids, as well as diuretics, antihypertensive medications and infection prophylaxis. Drug dosages need to be frequently adjusted in the light of laboratory results, such as cyclosporin levels. Most patients adjust well to the complex regime and are well rehabilitated.

Complications

Any signs of infection such as fever, or a new pulmonary infiltrate must be aggressively investigated to find the causative organism. As in any immunocompromised patient, a wide variety of organisms can cause infection. Particularly relevant to transplantation is cytomegalovirus (CMV), which classically presents as a fever about 1 month following transplantation. CMV may cause fatal infection if the patient is serologically CMV negative before surgery. If the

SURGICAL MANAGEMENT OF HEART DISEASE

heart is taken from a CMV positive donor, then prophylaxis is given, in the form CMV hyperimmune globulin. Similarly, toxoplasma negative patients will receive prophylaxis with co-trimoxazole.

About 15–20% of cardiac recipients die within the first year following transplantation. Most of these deaths occur within the first 3 months, and are caused by rejection of the heart or infection. The risk of rejection diminishes after this time, and the dosage of immunosuppressive drugs are cut back, thereby reducing the risk of infection and other side-effects, such as cyclosporin nephrotoxicity. The commonest cause of death beyond the first year is accelerated coronary atherosclerosis; a condition which is poorly understood, but which may be a form of chronic vascular rejection. In spite of these complications, the majority of heart transplant recipients become fully rehabilitated, and enjoy a good quality of life. Many return to full employment, and engage in active physical activity[43].

Heart transplantation is a rapidly changing subject. As well as continuing improvement in overall results as a consequence of increased experience and new immunosuppressive drugs, there are new developments occurring which will broaden the scope of transplantation in the future. Transplantation of the lungs, either singly or together with the heart, is now being performed: results are encouraging, but lung transplantation remains developmental at the present time.

Artificial hearts and left ventricular assist devices are being introduced as a means of sustaining acutely ill patients until a cardiac donor becomes available. These devices can save the lives of acutely ill patients in selected cases, but because the supply of donor hearts is limited, they will not significantly increase the total number of lives saved. However, within a few years, a permanently implantable, electrically powered left ventricular assist device will become available[46]. This will enable help to be given to patients who are unsuitable for transplantation, or who deteriorate before a donor heart becomes available. The potential application of permanent cardiac assist devices is great, with the associated implications for patient selection as well as the National Health care budget.

The cost of heart transplantation has been a controversial subject. However, with improving results and shortening hospital stays, the cost benefit ratio of heart transplantation has improved considerably over the last few years. The average cost of heart transplant in Britain today is about £17,000 for the first year's treatment, and about £4,000 a year thereafter[42]. This compares favourably with other accepted forms of therapy, such as renal dialysis, intravenous feeding and some cancer therapies.

In summary:

- heart transplantation is an accepted form of therapy, and gives good results;
- patients should be referred for transplantation before the onset of low cardiac output and multi-organ dysfunction;
- patients with myocarditis or acute cardiomyopathy who become haemodynamically compromised should be urgently considered for transplanting;
- transplant recipients have a good quality of life, but must be meticulous about their medical regime and follow-up appointments.

SUMMARY

Cardiac surgery has developed in phases, with different conditions becoming amenable to treatment as surgical techniques have progressed and results have improved. This sequence of development has been congenital surgery, valve surgery, coronary surgery and transplantation. The next phase will be the introduction of permanent assist devices.

With improving results, surgery has become recommended at earlier stages of the disease process. Most congenital surgery is now performed in infancy or early childhood, to avoid the onset of permanent myocardial damage and pulmonary vascular disease. Valve surgery is recommended before severe myocardial damage results, and coronary surgery is performed to prevent death from myocardial infarction, as well as for the symptomatic treatment of angina.

An awareness of the importance of the timing of surgical intervention is therefore extremely important. Appropriate investigation of the patient at an early stage of their disease is indicated. Nowadays this can often be done using non-invasive techniques, such as echocardiography, nuclear cardiology and exercise electrocardiography.

REFERENCES

1. Kirklin, J.W., Conti, V.R. and Blackstone, E.H. (1979). Prevention of myocardial damage during cardiac operation. *N. Engl. J. Med.*, **301**, 135-41
2. Foster, E.D., Fisher, L.D., Kaiser, G.C. and Myers, W.D. (1984). Principal investigators of CASS and associates: (1984). Comparison of operative mortality for initial and repeat coronary artery bypass grafting: The Coronary Artery Surgery Study (CASS) experience. *Ann. Thoracic Surg.*, **38**, 563–70
3. Chesebro, J.H., Clements, I.P., Fuster, V. *et al.* (1982). A platelet-inhibitor drug trial in coronary artery bypass operations. *N. Engl. J. Med.*, **307**, 73–8
4. Campeau, L., Lesperance, J., Hermann, J., Corbara, F., Grondin C.M. and Bourassa M.G. (1979). Loss of the improvement of angina between 1 and 4 years after aortocoronary bypass surgery. Correlations with changes in vein grafts and coronary arteries. *Circulation*, **60**, Suppl. I, 1–5
5. CASS principle investigators and associates: (1984). Myocardial infarction and mortality in the CASS study and randomised trial. *N. Engl. J. Med.*, **310**, 750
6. Myers, W.D., Gersh, B.J., Fisher, L.D., *et al.* (1987). Time to first myocardial infarction in patients with mild angina and three-vessel disease comparing medicine and early surgery: a CASS registry study of survival. *Ann. Thorac. Surg.*, **43**, 599
7. Varnauskas, E., and European Coronary Surgery Study Group. (1985). Survival, myocardial infarction, and employment status in a prospective randomised study of coronary bypass surgery. *Circulation*, **72** (Pt2), V, 90
8. Berg, R. Jr., Selinger, S.L., Leonard, J.J., Grunwald, R.P. and O'Grady, W.P. (1981). Immediate coronary artery bypass for acute evolving myocardial infarction. *J. Thorac. Cardiovasc. Surg.*, **81**, 493–47
9. Little, W.C. (1983). Thrombolytic therapy of acute myocardial infarction. *Curr. Probl. Cardiol.*, **8**, 4–47
10. European Study Group for Streptokinase in Acute Myocardial Infarction. (1979). Streptokinase in acute myocardial infarction. *N. Engl. J. Med.*, **301**, 797–802

11. Tector, A.I., Schmahl, T.M. and Canino, V.R. (1983). The internal mammary artery graft: The best choice for bypass of the left anterior descending coronary artery. *Circulation*, **68** (Pt2), V, 214–17
12. Kelsey, S.R., Mullin, S.M., Detre, K.M., Mitchell, H., Cowley, J., Greuntzig, A.R. and Kent, K.M. (1984). Effect of investigator experience on percutaneous transluminal coronary angioplasty. *Am. J. Cardiol.*, **53**, 12c–16c
13. Cowley, M.J., Dorros, G., Kelsey S.F., Van Raden M. and Detre K.M. (1984). Acute coronary events associated with percutaneous transluminal coronary angioplasty. *Am. J. Cardiol.*, **53**, 12c–16c
14. Holmes, D.R. Jr., Viletstra, R.E., Smith, H.C., *et al.* (1984). Restenosis after percutaneous transluminal coronary angioplasty (PTCA): A report from the PTCA registry of the National Heart, Lung, and Blood Institute. *Am. J. Cardiol.*, **53**, 77c–81c
15. Williams, D.C., Greuntzig, A.R., Kent, K.M., Kelsey, S.F. and To T. (1984). Efficiency of repeat percutaneous transluminal coronary angioplasty on stenosis. *Am. J. Cardiol.*, **53**, 32c–35c
16. Schaff, H.V., Orzulak, T., Gersh, B.J., Piehler, J.M., Puga, F.J., Danielson, G.K. and Pluth, J.R. (1983). The morbidity and mortality of reoperation for coronary artery disease, and analysis of late results with use of actuarial estimate of event-free survival. *J. Thorac. Cardiovasc. Surg.*, **85**, 508–15
17. Cheitlin, M.D. (1987). The timing of surgery in mitral and aortic valve disease. *Curr. Probl. Cardiol.*, **12**, 69–149
18. Richards, K.L. (1985). Doppler echocardiography in diagnosis and quantification of valvular heart disease. *Curr. Probl. Cardiol.*, **10**, 3–49
19. Commerford, P.J., Hastie, T. and Beck, W. (1982). Closed mitral valvotomy: actuarial analysis of results in 654 patients over 12 years, and analysis of perioperative predictions of long-term survival. *Ann. Thorac. Surg.*, **33**, 473–9
20. Grollier, G., Hutet, B., Foucault, J.P. and Potier, J.C. (1987). Percutaneous mitral valvotomy in rheumatic mitral stenosis: a new approach. *Br. Heart J.*, **33**, 473–9
21. Sethia, B., Turner, M.A., Lewis, S., Rodger, R.A. and Bain, W.H. (1986). Fourteen years experience with the Bjork–Shiley tilting disk prosthesis. *J. Thorac. Cardiovasc. Surg.*, **91**, 350–61
22. Lindblom, D. (1988). Long-term clinical results after mitral valve replacement with the Bjork–Shiley prosthesis. *J. Thorac. Cardiovasc. Surg.*, **95**, 321–33
23. Duncan, J.M., Cooley, D.A., Reul, G.J., *et al.* (1986). Durability and low thrombogenicity of the St Jude Medical Valve at 5 year follow-up. *Ann. Thorac. Surg.*, **42**, 500–5
24. Pass, H.I., Sade, R.M., Crawford, F.A., and Hohm, A.R. (1984). Cardiac valve prosthesis in children without anticoagulation. *J. Thorac. Cardiovasc. Surg.*, **87**, 832

25. Jamusz, M.T., Jamieson, W.R., Allen, P., et al. (1982). Experience with the Carpentier–Edwards porcine valve prosthesis in 700 patients. *Ann. Thorac. Surg.*, **34**, 625–33
26. Bolooki, H., Kaiser, G.A., Mallon, S.M. and Palatinos, G.M. (1986). Comparison of long-term results of Carpentier–Edwards and Hancock bioprosthetic valves. *Ann. Thorac. Surg.*, **42**, 494–9
27. Reul, G.J., Cooley, D.A. and Duncan, J.M. (1985). Valve failure with the Ionescu–Shiley bovine pericardial bioprosthesis: analysis of 2680 patients. *J. Vasc. Surg.*, **2**, 192–206
28. Hammond, G.L., Geha, A.S., Kopf, G.S. and Hashim, S.W. (1987). Biological versus mechanical valves. Analysis of 1,116 valves inserted in 1,012 adult patients with a 4,818 patient–year and a 5,,327 valve-year follow up. *J. Thorac. Cardiovasc. Surg.*, **93**, 182–98
29. Penta, A., Qureschi, S., Radley-Smith, R. and Yacoub, M.H. (1984). Patient status 10 or more years after fresh homograft replacement of the aortic valve. *Circulation*, **70**, (Suppl I), I182–I186
30. McGoon, D.C. (1960). Repair of mitral insufficiency due to ruptured chordae tendinae. *J. Thorac. Cardiovasc. Surg.*, **39**, 357
31. Carpentier, A., Deloche, A., Dauptin, J., et al. (1971). A new reconstructive operation for correction of mitral and tricuspid insufficiency. *J. Thorac. Cardiovasc. Surg.*, **61**, 1–13
32. Orsulak, T.A., Schaff, H.V., Danielson, G.K., et al. (1985). Mitral regurgitation due to ruptured chordae tendinae. *J. Thorac. Cardiovasc. Surg.*, **89**, 491–8
33. Angell, W.W., Oury, J.H. and Shah, P. (1987). A comparison of replacement and reconstruction in patients with mitral regurgitation. *J. Thorac. Cardiovasc. Surg.*, **93**, 665–74
34. Cohn, L.H., Kowalker, W., Bhatia, S., DiSesa, V.J., St. John-Sutton, M., Shemin, R.J. and Collins, J.J. (1988). Comparative morbidity of mitral valve repair versus replacement for mitral regurgitation with and without coronary artery disease. *Ann. Thorac. Surg.*, **45**, 284–90
35. King, R.M., Pluth, J.R. and Giuliani, E.R. (1986). Mechanical decalcification of the aortic valve. *Ann. Thorac. Surg.*, **42**, 269–72
36. Ross, R. Jr. (1985). Afterload mismatch in aortic and mitral valve disease: implications for surgical therapy. *J. Am. Coll. Cardiol.*, **5**, 811–26
37. Nishimura, R.A., McGoon, M.D., Schaff, H.V. and Giuliani, E.R. (1988). Chronic aortic regurgitation: indications for operation. *Mayo Clin. Proc.*, **63**, 270–21
38. Fioretti, P., Roelandt, J., Bos, R.J., Meltzer, R.S., Van Hoogenhijze, D., Semys, P.W., Nauta, J. and Hugenholtz, P.G. (1983). Echocardiography in chronic aortic insufficiency: is valve replacement too late when left ventricular end systolic dimension reaches 55 mm? *Circulation*, **67**, 216–21
39. Barnard, C.N. (1967). The operation. *S. Afr. Med. J.*, **41**, 1271–6

40. Caves, P.K., Stinson, E.B., Billingham, M.E., Rider, A.K. and Shumway, N.E. (1973). Diagnosis of human cardiac allograft rejection by serial cardiac biopsy. *J. Thorac. Cardiovasc. Surg.*, **66**, 461-6
41. Oyer, P.E., Stinson, E.B., Jamieson, S.W., *et al*. (1982). One year experience with cyclosporin A in clinical heart transplantation. *J. Heart Transplant.*, 285-95
42. Buxton, M., Acheson, R.M., Caine, M., Gibson, S. and O'Brien, B. (1985). Costs and benefits of heart transplantation programmes at Harefield and Papworth Hospitals. Research Report No. 12 (Brunel Report) H.M.S.O.
43. Schroeder, J.S. and Hunt, S. (1987). Cardiac transplantation, update 1987. *J. Am. Med. Assoc.*, **258**, 3142-5
44. Stevenson, L.W., Fowler, M.B., Schroeder, J.S., Stevenson, W.G., Dracup, K.A. and Ford, V. (1987). Poor survival of patients with idiopathic cardiomyopathy considered too well for transplantation. *Am. J. Med.*, **83**, 871-6
45. Conference of the Medical Royal Colleges and their faculties in the United Kingdom: Diagnosis of brain death. *Br. Med. J.*, **2**, 1187-8
46. McGregor, G.G.A. (1987). Prospects for the artificial heart. In Sobel, Julian, Huggenholtz, (eds). *Perspectives in Cardiology*. (London: Current Medical Literature)

Index

acetylcholine activity in normal
  conditions, 5
aetiology of heart failure, *see* cause
afterload, 2–3
  increased, 8, 39–40
age
  coronary artery bypass grafting
    indications related to, 64
  heart transplantation indications
    related to, 78
aldosterone (in regulation of cardiac
    function)
  in heart failure, 12
  in normal conditions, 6, 7
α-receptors
  in heart failure, 11
  in normal conditions, 5
amiloride, in combined diuretic
    therapy, 46
aminophylline, in acute left
    ventricular failure management,
    54
angina
  management, 59–66 *passim*
  recurrent, 61, 65
angioplasty
  coronary occlusion following, 63
  percutaneous transluminal
    coronary, 64–5
  coronary artery bypass grafting
    compared with, 65
angiotensin II (in regulation of
    cardiac function)
  in heart failure, 12
  in normal conditions, 6, 7
angiotensin converting enzyme
  (ACE) inhibitors, 48–9, 50
  diuretic therapy with the addition
    of, 47
  side-effects, 49
aortic valve
  chronic disease, causes, 67
  regurgitation, 75–6
  repair, 73
  stenosis, 74
apex beat in left ventricular failure, 23
arrhythmias, 9–10
arterial disease, increase resistance
  due to, increased afterload
  caused by, 8
artificial hearts, 81
artificial valves, 69–72
asthma, cardiac and bronchial,
  differentiation, 24
atrial natriuretic factor, 7–8
autonomic nervous system (in
  regulation of cardiac function),
  see also parasympathetic
  nervous system; sympathetic
  nervous system
  in heart failure, 11
  in normal conditions, 5–6

backward failure, 19–20
bendrofluazide, in chronic heart
  failure management, 41

INDEX

β-receptors
  in heart failure, 11
  in normal conditions, 5
biological valves, 70–2
biopsies, endomyocardial/cardiac, 33
  for rejection diagnosis, 77, 80
Bjork–Shiley valve, 69, 70
blood pressure in left ventricular
    failure, 23
blood volume (circulating),
    increased/excessive, 18
  increased preload caused by, 8
boot-shaped heart, 28, 29
bovine pericardium, valves made
    from, 71
breathlessness
  in left ventricular failure, 20
  in right ventricular failure, 24

cachexia, in right ventricular failure,
    26–7
calcium ions in muscle contraction, 6
captopril, 30–1
  diuretic therapy with the addition
    of, 47
  enalapril v., 48–9
  side-effects, 49
carbon, pyrolite, valves made of,
    69–70
cardiovascular signs
  in left ventricular failure, 22–3
  in right ventricular failure, 26
catheterization, cardiac, 32–3
  coronary occlusion following, 63
  of left side of heart, 32
  of potential heart transplant
    recipients, 78–9
  of right side of heart, 32–3
  in valve disease, 68
causes of heart failure, 8, 17–20, 37–8
  correctable, 37
chest X-ray, 28–30
chronic heart failure, management,
    38–53

summary of, 52
classification of heart failure, 21–4
closed heart surgery with valve
    disease, 68
compensatory mechanisms in heart
    failure, 10–12, 39–40
congestive heart failure, ambiguous
    meaning, 12–13
congestive manifestations of heart
    failure, 14–15
contraction, myocardial/cardiac
  normal, 3, 6
  reduced, causes, 9
coronary angioplasty, percutaneous
    transluminal, *see* angioplasty
coronary artery
  anatomy, 61–2
  disease affecting all three
    branches, 62
  disease affecting left anterior
    descending, 62, 64
  occlusion following cardiac
    catheterization or angioplasty,
    63
  surgery, 59–63
    percutaneous transluminal
      coronary angioplasty compared
      with, 65
    symptomatic benefits, 61
cough, ACE inhibitor-related, 49
creatinine, blood urea/serum, in right
    ventricular failure, 27
cytomegalovirus infection,
    post-cardiac transplantation,
    80–1

death, *see also* terminal heart failure
  cardiac transplant-related, 81
  coronary artery bypass
    graft-related, 60
  from myocardial infarction, 60, 62
  in heart failure, 55
definitions of heart failure, 1, 17
diabetes, heart transplantation in, 78

diagnosis of heart failure, 36–8
diamorphine
   in acute left ventricular failure management, 53–4
   in terminal left ventricular failure management, 55
digoxin
   in chronic heart failure therapy, 50–3
   prescription, 50–3
   role, 50
   toxicity, symptoms, 51
dilatation, cardiac, as a compensatory mechanisms in heart failure, 10–11
diuretics
   in acute left ventricular failure management, 53
   in chronic heart failure management, 41–7, 52
      combined, 45–6
      monitoring of responses to, 46–7
      vasodilators added with, 47
   classes, 41, *see also specific classes*
dobutamine therapy, 53
donors, cardiac, 79
dopamine therapy, 53
drugs, 38–54
   in acute left ventricular failure management, 53–4
   in chronic heart failure management, 38–53
      aims, 38–9
      principles, 39–40
Duramedic valve, 69–70
dysrhythmias, 9–10

echocardiography, 31
   in valve disease, 68, 72
electrocardiography, 31
electrolytes, serum, in heart failure, 27
enalapril, 48–9
   captopril v., 48–9
   side-effects, 49

endomyocardial biopsy, *see* biopsies
exacerbating factors in heart failure, 37

fatigue on effort
   in left ventricular failure, 22
   in right ventricular failure, 24
forward failure, 19–20
Frank–Starling Law, 2, 4
   in heart failure, 10–11
frusemide, 42–3
   ACE inhibitors added with, 47
   in acute left ventricular failure management, 53

gallop rhythm, 14
gastrointestinal symptoms in right ventricular failure, 24
heart
   artificial, 81
   biopsies, *see* biopsies
   dilatation, as a compensatory mechanisms in heart failure, 10–11, 39–40
   donors, 79
   function
      compensatory mechanisms in disease, 10–12, 39–40
      major factors influencing, 2–3
      normal regulation, 3–8
   hypertrophy, 12
   murmurs, in left ventricular failure, 23
   output, *see* output
   physiology, normal, 1–3
   radiology, 50
   recipients, assessment, 78–9
   sounds, in left ventricular failure, 23
   transplantation, *see* transplantation
hepatomegaly in right ventricular failure, 26
hormonal mechanisms, *see* neurohormonal mechanisms

INDEX

hydralazine, isosorbide dinitrate plus, 49–50
hypertrophy, cardiac, 12
hypokalaemia, diuretic-induced, 43–5
  prevention and correction, 44–5
hypotension, ACE inhibitor-related, 49

immunocompromised cardiac transplant patients, infection in, 80–1
infarction, myocardial, *see* myocardial infarction
infection, post-cardiac transplantation, 80–1
inotropic agents, 50–3
  in chronic heart failure management, 40
intrinsic disease, heart failure caused by, 17–18
investigations in heart failure, 27–33, *see also specific techniques*
Ionescu–Shiley valve, 71
ischaemic heart disease, surgery, 58–66
isosorbide dinitrate, hydralazine plus, 49–50
isotope (radio-) studies, 32

laboratory tests, 27–8
left heart failure, *see also* ventricular failure
  monitoring responses to drug therapy, 46
  symptoms and signs, 39
left-to-right heart shunting, increased preload caused by, 8
liver
  functional tests, 27–8
  in right ventricular failure, 26
loop diuretics, 41, 42–3
  side-effects, 42, 43
  thiazide advantages over, 42
lungs, *see also entries under* pulmonary

  in left ventricular failure, 23
  radiology, 28
  in right ventricular failure, 26–7

mammary artery, internal, coronary bypass grafting employing, 64
mechanical valves, 69–70, 71–2
mental symptoms in left ventricular failure, 22
metabolic demands on heart, increased, 18
mitral valve
  regurgitation, 14, 72, 74–5
    acute, causes, 67
  repair, 72
  stenosis, 73–4
  valvotomy, closed, 68–9
mortality, *see* death
murmurs, in left ventricular failure, 23
myocardial biopsy, *see* biopsies
myocardial contraction, *see* contraction
myocardial disease, terminal, 76–82
myocardial infarction, 62, 63
  acute, 63, 66
  complications, 66
  death from, 60, 62
  role of surgery following, 63, 66
myocardial revascularization, 59–66

neck veins in right ventricular failure, 26
neurohormonal mechanisms (in regulation of cardiac function)
  in heart failure, 12
  in normal conditions, 6–8
noradrenaline activity in normal conditions, 5

oedema
  in heart failure, 26, 36
    pulmonary, radiography, 28, 30
  other causes, 36
output, cardiac, 1

low, 13

parasympathetic nervous system in regulation of cardiac function, 5
pericardium, bovine, valves made from, 71
physiological regulation of cardiac function, normal, 4
physiology, heart, normal, 1–3
porcine valves, 70–1
potassium problems, diuretic-related, 43–5
potassium-sparing diuretics, 41, 43
  in combined diuretic therapy, 44
prazosin, 30
precipitating factors in heart failure, 19, 38
preload, 2
  increased, 8, 39–40
prosthetic devices, *see entries under* artificial
pulmonary oedema, radiography, 28, 30
pulmonary vascular resistance measurement in potential heart transplant recipients, 78–9
pyrolite carbon, valves made of, 69–70

radiology, 28–30
radionuclide/radio-isotope studies, 32
recipients of heart transplants, assessment, 78–9
rejection diagnosis, cardiac biopsies for, 77, 80
renin–angiotensin–aldosterone system (in regulation of cardiac function)
  in heart failure, 12
  in normal conditions, 6, 7
resistance, increased, heart failure caused by, 18
rheumatic heart disease, valvular involvement in, 66–7
rhythm

disorders, 9–10, *see also specific disorders*
gallop, 14
right heart failure, *see also* ventricular failure
  monitoring responses to drug therapy in, 46
  symptoms and signs, 39

St Jude valve, 69–70
saphenous vein, long, grafts employing, 59–60
  alternatives to, 64
  thrombosis with, 61
shunting, left-to-right (heart), increased preload caused by, 8
signs (of heart failure)
  of left ventricular failure, 14–15, 22–3
  physical, 39
  of right ventricular failure, 15, 25, 26–7
sinus rhythm, digoxin in management of, 50
sounds, heart, in left ventricular failure, 23
spironolactone, 45
  in combined diuretic therapy, 45–6
Starling's Law, *see* Frank–Starling Law
Starr–Edwards valve, 69, 70
surgery, 57–83
  in terminal heart failure, 54, 76–82
sympathetic nervous system (in regulation of cardiac function)
  in normal conditions, 5
  stimulation/overactivity, 11, 13–14
    clinical features, 13–14
symptoms (of heart failure), 39
  in left ventricular failure, 20–2
  in right ventricular failure, 24–6

tachycardias/tachydysrhythmias, 9, 10

INDEX

technetium, radio-isotope studies with, 32
terminal heart failure, management, 54–5, 76–82, *see also* death
  surgical, 54, 76–82
thallium, radio-isotope studies with, 32
thiazides
  in chronic heart failure management, 41–2
  side-effects, 42, 43
thrombolytic therapy in acute myocardial infarction, 63
thrombosis of vein grafts, 61
transplantation, heart, 54, 76–82
  complications, 80–1
  contraindications, 78
  cost, 82
  donors, 79
  indications, 77–8
  postoperative course, 80
  recipients, assessment, 78–9
  in terminal heart disease, 54, 76–82
triamterene, in combined diuretic therapy, 46
tricuspid valve disease, 66
triple vessel disease, 62

urinary signs and symptoms, 27
  in left ventricular failure, 22

valves, *see also specific valves*
  artificial/prosthetic, 69–72
  diseased, 66–76
    early surgery for, indications, 67
    increased preload caused by, 8
  repair, 72–3
vasoconstriction, angiotensin II-mediated, 6

vasodilators, 48–50, 54
  in acute left ventricular failure management, 54
  in chronic heart failure, 48–50, 52
  diuretic therapy with the addition of, 47
  regimen choices, 50
ventricles
  increased resistance encountered by, 18
  obstruction to outflow of, increased afterload caused by, 8
ventricular assist devices, left, 81
ventricular enlargement, left, radiological investigation, 28, 29
ventricular failure, 20–7
  left, 14–15, 20–3
    acute, management, 53
    diagnosis, 36
    signs/manifestations, 14–15, 22–3
    symptoms, 20–2
    terminal/death, 55
  right, 15, 24–7
    signs/manifestations, 15, 25, 26–7
    symptoms, 24–6
ventricular filling, impaired, 9
ventricular function, left, impaired, 9
  patients with angina and, surgery for, 63–4
volume, blood, *see* blood volume

weighing, drug therapy responses monitored via, in right heart failure, 28
wheezing in left ventricular failure, 21
workload, excessive, heart failure caused by, 18–19

X-ray, chest, 28–30